HOMEBIRTH HANDBOOK

How to have your baby calmly and safely at home

ANNIE FRANCIS

1 3 5 7 9 10 8 6 4 2

Vermilion, an imprint of Ebury Publishing,
20 Vauxhall Bridge Road,
London SW1 V 2SA

Vermilion is part of the Penguin Random House group of companies
whose addresses can be found at global.penguinrandomhouse.com

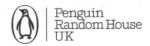

Penguin
Random House
UK

First published in the United Kingdom by Vermilion in 2016

www.penguin.co.uk

A CIP catalogue record for this book is available from the British Library

ISBN 9781785040245

Printed and bound in Great Britain by Clays Ltd, St Ives PLC

Penguin Random House is committed to a sustainable future for our
business, our readers and our planet. This book is made from Forest
Stewardship Council® certified paper.

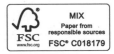

The information in this book has been compiled by way of general guidance
in relation to the specific subjects addressed, but is not a substitute and
not to be relied on for medical, healthcare, pharmaceutical or other
professional advice on specific circumstances and in specific locations. So
far as the author is aware the information given is correct and up to date
as at November 2014. Practice, laws and regulations all change, and the
reader should obtain up to date professional advice on any such issues. The
author and publishers disclaim, as far as the law allows, any liability arising
directly or indirectly from the use, or misuse, of the information contained
in this book.

Contents

Preface – Cathy Warwick, CBE, Chief Executive of the Royal College of Midwives

This book is a delight. It is beautifully written, accessible and treats its readers with the greatest respect, presenting a full, considered and honest account of home birth. The author, Annie Francis, is a busy midwife for whom I have the greatest admiration. In this book her passion for midwifery and her respect for women shine through as she helps them and their partners think about the possibility of choosing a home birth and why it is that home birth, despite the evidence that supports it as a safe choice for women to make, is so uncommon in our society today.

Annie does not hesitate to use her own childbirth history and her own experience as a midwife to illustrate her writing. This, along with her references to other experts, to relevant literature and to the stories of other women has the effect of making her book feel very authentic. This is neither a dense academic tome nor a very lightweight summary of information. Rather it is an enjoyable, engaging and informative read which recognises that for many women making the important decision as to where to give birth is one that requires a lot of thought and a much broader understanding of the issues than is generally presented.

The book however is not merely about making the choice of home birth – it is also about the practicalities of birthing at home, should that choice be made, and in this respect Annie does an excellent job of interweaving the what with the why. This is what I mean by treating readers with respect. Annie recognises that it isn't enough to simply tell women what might happen and how they therefore can best cope. Adding in more detailed explanation, whether that is about the way the uterus works or how the different stages of labour unfold, makes it all make so much more sense.

Annie is also completely honest with her reader. Not every woman choosing to birth at home will actually do so. The possibility of transfer in labour and of complications arising is as clearly outlined as any other aspect of the subject and again in a way which I am sure can only be of the greatest help to women and their partners.

The book is presented in three parts – part 1: 'Planning your Home Birth', part 2: 'Birth Stories' and part 3: 'The History and Politics Underpinning Modern Childbirth' – and each could be read separately. However, Annie's writing is such that they feel woven together each part informing the other and each building on the other to create the total, very compelling picture that this book presents to us.

As a midwife of many years myself, with experience of supporting women to make their own informed choice of place of birth and of supporting many women to birth at home, I welcome this book. Ultimately what is critical is that women make choices with which they feel comfortable and safe but it is hard for them to do that without having easy access to information which is presented in an unbiased and engaging way by someone with real-life experience. This is the essence of Annie's book.

Foreword – Lily Cole, mother and actor

You can't really plan birth. Every woman's experience is different and unexpected. I aimed for a home birth with an open mind about going to hospital, and I ended up getting the two. Both parts of the experience were extraordinary in different ways.

When I found out I was pregnant, I called Annie Francis – Annie – mother of four, my friend's mother, independent midwife and the founder of the pioneering organisation Neighbourhood Midwives. Annie works on the premise that women are amazing creatures whose biological wisdom knows how to birth a baby. She made me feel confident and able to have the birth my partner and I wanted. I trusted her implicitly. Throughout my pregnancy and the postnatal period, Annie went from being my friend's mother, to my midwife, to my friend, to eventually becoming my daughter's godmother.

Having my baby girl was the most important thing I have done since my own birth. It was the second birth of me. I am so glad my daughter's first experience of life – of that transition from womb to world – was a positive and gentle one. Wylde was born at home, with two midwives present (Annie Francis and Rae Vrdoljak) alongside my partner and me. It was 4am and the world was quiet outside. There were no drugs in her system. I think the experience we had together in those first moments has shaped the months that have followed, and potentially informed our daughter's calm and fearless spirit.

It seems to me that our society has medicalised and institutionalised birth over the past few decades. Women have been discouraged from having their babies naturally at home, in spite of the positive evidence in favour of it. Although I had to transfer to hospital after the birth, a home birth meant I got to bring my little girl into the world in an intimate, private, sacred way. And I got to witness what my body is capable of.

I always knew that transfer to hospital was a possibility. Indeed, the fact that I live close to one made having a home birth feel safe and wise. We were given a brilliant insight into how the natural and medical worlds can meet and complement each other. After the birth, I had a complication with my placenta, so Annie called an ambulance and within an hour I was in a hospital. I stayed in for two days, receiving fantastic care, before being discharged home again.

Annie combines spirituality with pragmatism. She is the biggest advocate of home births, but also the biggest advocate of hospitals when necessary. She guided me through this experience with real focus and a strong instinct. I felt supported and empowered and I would recommend her insights in a heartbeat.

Aim for the experience that feels right for you. Do your research, and make an informed decision regarding how you would like the birth to happen, bearing in mind no birth can be totally planned. Make a decision that is not based on fear. Hire a doula or independent midwife if you can. Read this book. Believe in your body. However you do it, believe that birth can be a positive and empowering experience.

Lily Cole

Introduction

B eing born is an experience that all living creatures have in
common. Whatever the unique details of our own birth,
each one of us has been through it and the manner of our birth
can shape our lives forever. The act of giving birth is often a
seminal moment in a woman's life, which changes and redefines
her and can be an opportunity for personal growth because of
the often intense physical and psychological challenges it may
present. Labour and birth might be remembered as a traumatic
event that can cause lifelong pain and suffering, both physically
and emotionally, or as a positive and empowering episode in
one's life, the memory of which can be revisited to give strength
in times of difficulty. Because it has this ability to affect our lives
so profoundly, I really believe that, as women, we need to actively
take responsibility for the planning and preparation for labour
and birth – including the decision about where we choose to be –
rather than allow that decision to be made for us, often by default.

I have four children, three of whom were born at home, and
all my labours and births were relatively easy (despite the fact
that two were breech) in terms of the physical act of giving
birth. For me, it was the emotional and psychological process
involved that fundamentally changed me as a person. I am a
midwife today because of how deeply the births of my children
have impacted on my life.

Although I am trained in and familiar with using obstetric equipment and following hospital procedures, protocols and policies, I don't see myself as a 'high-tech' midwife – a bustling labour ward with its bright lights and machinery is simply not an environment where I enjoy working. For me, all those monitors beeping away (not to mention the excessive paperwork and bureaucracy that come with a hospital setting) are a distraction, preventing me from giving my full attention to the individual person in my care. Put me in a quiet, comfortable space with a woman in labour at home, and I am happy to sit there for hours, witnessing her power and marvelling as the wonder of birth unfolds. Of course, this is not without great effort on the part of the mother – and it is even a struggle for her at times – but when she finally meets her baby, she is rewarded with an oxytocin high (women get a big surge of this so-called 'love hormone' immediately after the birth), and the bonus of being able to relax in her own bed.

Although I have worked in the National Health Service (NHS), most of my experience gained over the past 18 years or so of midwifery practice has been in independent practice doing mostly home births. Actually, I think home is probably in my DNA (I was the only one of six children to be born there) as it instinctively feels like a good place to labour in – somewhere you can relax properly, switch off the thinking, planning part of your brain and go into 'the zone' with peace and privacy in order to have your baby with the minimum of intervention.

While acknowledging that obstetric units have done a lot in recent years to improve the birthing environment, the truth is that having your baby at home is so much more than just being in 'home-like' surroundings. It is your space, your territory and no amount of nice furniture or pictures on the wall can replace that. There is also something deeply satisfying about having a bath afterwards in your own bathroom and then getting into your own bed with your new baby, knowing that you don't need to go anywhere else and can just relax into getting to know each other.

If we are to make home birth a realistic choice for many more women, we need to revisit the language we use around birth, especially the implication that women are 'not allowed' to make certain choices. The system needs to change to a much more open-minded approach, with women being supported to find the path that feels right for them.

To do that, we need to change the current status quo, moving from providing a restrictive 'menu' of what is available, to facilitating and supporting women to access different options. The service must work in genuine partnership with women, enabling them, through effective information sharing, to become much more proactive in all the decisions about their care. Of course, this doesn't just apply to home birth – feeling more 'in charge' of what happens to them will empower all women, wherever they wish to have their baby.

Making home birth a genuine and realistic choice, with comprehensive and balanced information about the risks and benefits, will flow from a change in attitude from healthcare professionals and a more equal approach to information sharing, rather than just information giving.

I have no doubt that these changes are coming, because a fundamental reform and rethink of the system is necessary and long overdue. And, as the benefits of home birth gradually become more widely appreciated, my hope is that this book will play its own small part in promoting the concept. By providing lots of ideas for the practical, psychological and physical preparation for home birth, my aim is to help you achieve a straightforward, safe and positive experience – all within the comfort and security of your own home.

The book is divided into three parts. Part 1 is all about the actual planning involved when choosing a home birth, including a practical guide to the preparation and 'equipment' needed. My aim is to help you think through how you can best prepare yourself during the months of pregnancy to be ready – mentally and physically – for the challenge of labour and the birth of your baby. I have made some suggestions about what you can do to improve your chances of successfully having your baby at home but would stress that it is important to keep an open mind and to be able to accept that, despite your best efforts, things don't always go according to plan. It's not a failure to change your mind or your plans; it's a sensible and mature response to life's unexpected turn of events, and your birth experience can and should be a positive one wherever it takes place.

I also explore the concept of risk and safety as currently defined within the 'risk management' approach of our maternity services and ask whether it is an effective way of assessing an individual woman's level of risk in the context of her own unique set of circumstances. How do you personally decide what safety means to you and how do you balance or mitigate the specific element of 'risk' that may be present in your own situation?

Part 2 comprises stories of birth. They have been sent in from across the country and cover a range of experiences. Some are more challenging than others but all are inspirational and I hope you will enjoy reading them as much as I have.

Part 3 is a more in-depth exploration of some of the history and politics of birth that underpin the thinking and reasons for choosing a home birth today. I've gone back briefly through past millennia to explore what we know about how women have given birth in the past and to challenge the myth that human females have some sort of design fault. Given the current world population and the complete domination of our species across the planet, I would dispute the idea that once we stood up on two legs instead of four, we compromised our physical ability to give birth to our offspring. I've included the most recent theory about metabolic limits and what it tells us about why human infants are born when they are, completely helpless and needing total care and attention.

I then look at the more recent history of the maternity services in the United Kingdom, including how the medical model of childbirth came to dominate policy and practice. Within that context, I revisit the work of Marjorie Tew, whose detailed analysis of the official maternity data in the 1980s and 1990s challenged the established and widely held belief that birth in hospital must always be safer than at home. I read her book, *Safer Childbirth? A Critical History of Maternity Care*,[1] while I was a student midwife and was an immediate and lifelong fan!

It's also worth saying that there are lots of related areas that this book doesn't cover, partly because they are already written about elsewhere, and in much greater depth and detail than I could ever do, but also because it seems sensible just to focus on what I know and love.

So, if you are pregnant and beginning to think about what decisions to make about how and where you have your baby, my advice is to give it proper consideration because I believe it really does matter. It seems to me that something so fundamental as where to bring your baby into the world should be thought through carefully, whatever the conclusions you reach. If you are reading this book because you are thinking, however vaguely, about staying at home to have your baby, I hope that it will provide the answers to any questions you may have and will give you plenty of food for thought about the benefits of a home birth as well as offering a balanced view of the risks associated with the different options you have available.

Finally, I wish you a positive and fulfilling birth experience, wherever you choose – or need – to be!

Annie Francis

PART I

Planning Your Home Birth

The Context for Contemporary Home Birth

When contemplating making an important choice in life, most of us will seek the advice of people we trust and use the experiences of our closest friends and family to inform our decisions. Choosing where to have your baby is no different in some respects, but because it is intensely personal in nature and involves the wellbeing of a third person who has no say in the matter, it may be harder to remain objective and dispassionate about the options, especially when everyone you ask will usually have, and feel happy to voice, a very strong opinion about what you should do.

My suggestion, therefore, is that it might be helpful when thinking through your preferences and about the choices that are right for you, to consider them in the wider context of human birth through the ages. In Part 3 I go into more detail about this, but for now it is useful to bear in mind that modern ideas about how women cope with labour change frequently and are not set in stone.

Indeed, it is important to remember that women have been successfully giving birth, with little or no intervention, for countless generations prior to the more recent developments in technological birth in the developed world. However, a cursory read through the caesarean section (a surgical procedure to deliver the baby by cutting through the mother's abdomen and uterus) rates of different countries might lead you to pause and seriously question this fact. According to the World Health Organization for example, Brazil has a caesarean section rate of 80–90 per cent in the private sector and 55 per cent nationally, with more and more women reportedly viewing natural birth as primitive, ugly and inconvenient. Closer to home, Italy has a caesarean section rate of almost 40 per cent, and, at the other end of the scale, the Netherlands has only 16 per cent.[2] In contrast, home birth rates in the Netherlands are 20 per cent (2013), while they are 2.3 per cent in the United Kingdom and 0.86 per cent in the United States (2012).[3]

What these different figures illustrate is that the rates of intervention and home birth in different countries have less to do with individual women and their ability to give birth than with the health system and prevailing culture within a particular country.

The reason why this matters is that, when considering your own personal preferences, it can be immensely empowering and liberating to realise that there is plenty you can do as an individual to increase the likelihood of achieving the outcome you want. By first acknowledging the current dominant practices and behaviours in our culture, you make possible the next step, which is to actively decide not to simply follow the status quo but to choose to do things differently.

One example is your level of fitness. Speaking very generally, we have become used to a more sedentary lifestyle in the West and are less naturally fit than our more nomadic hunter-gatherer ancestors were. This can impact on our ability and stamina to remain active in labour and work with our babies to help them negotiate their journey through the pelvis with the minimum of difficulty. Therefore, you have to proactively choose to take exercise and consciously make it a part of your regular regime – a habit it will do no harm to maintain throughout your life but one that can easily be introduced when you first discover you are expecting a baby – or at least once you are over the worst of any morning sickness!

You may be surprised to learn that having a 'birth partner' to help support and guide you through labour and birth is also an important part of the cultural and evolutionary aspects of birth. Nowadays most of us will have an expectation that our partner (usually the father of the baby) will be there at the birth, but this hasn't always been the case and need not necessarily be so for you – or indeed be your only support. It is worth spending some time considering who else you might want to have with you during labour. Then, once you have decided, meeting together and agreeing what their role(s) will be is an important part of your planning. There is a reason why, unlike most other mammals, we don't tend to do birth on our own. I explore this further in Part 3, because understanding the roots of that need is all part of the preparation and sense of control we can exert over the process.

The United Kingdom is somewhat unusual in that we still have a healthy and vibrant midwifery profession. Women expect to be cared for by midwives during their pregnancy and understand that midwives will still, by and large, be the person delivering their baby, even though doctors will be involved if or when they are needed. When you book in for your maternity care, it will generally be a midwife you meet first, although, under the current NHS, you are unlikely to have only one midwife caring for you all the way through your pregnancy.

Because it is definitely helpful – and preferable – to know who your midwife will be at the birth, it is worth bearing in mind that one of the best ways of improving your chances of meeting and getting to know a small group of midwives who will then look after you all the way through your pregnancy, is to request a home birth and, one hopes, be assigned to a home birth or caseload team (*see* page 30) in your area. Forging a strong and mutually respectful relationship with one or two midwives can, in my opinion, improve your chances of experiencing a positive and enjoyable pregnancy and can be a crucial ingredient in the successful outcome of your planned home birth.

The risk versus safety debate

When contemplating whether or not to stay at home to have your baby, you need to have an honest and open debate with yourself and with your partner about the question of risk and safety as they are currently understood in relation to childbirth. This is because these are the two areas most likely to come up again and again, especially if you are quite open about sharing with others that your preferred place of birth is at home. 'Isn't it too risky?' and 'Is it safe?' are, given the culture of fear that now surrounds birth, the most common concerns that your friends and family are likely to voice.

And it is highly probable that one of the thoughts, however fleeting, that will pass through your mind from time to time throughout your pregnancy will be along the lines of 'Will my baby be okay?', 'What if something happens to him/her during the birth?' and 'What if something happens to me?'

Whatever your situation and whoever you are, these thoughts are completely normal. Having a baby is one of those events that is right up there in the top ten 'stressful/life-changing/momentous/frightening/intense/exciting/joyful' (insert which ones apply to you) situations and, as such, will demand a lot of focus and concentration. Perhaps these thoughts about the risk – potential or otherwise – to our own or our baby's health and survival are part of our coping mechanisms; it is also important that we take this role seriously because growing, birthing and then taking responsibility for another human being is strongly linked to the continuance and survival of our species.

Linked to these thoughts and feelings is the development over time of an increasingly strong protective instinct that we feel towards our growing babies, which often starts with the pregnancy and peaks with, or soon after, the birth. This instinct can contribute to at least some of the moments of anxiety or disquiet you may have about the risks your baby might face in his or her journey out into the world. Of course, this maternal instinct to protect and defend our offspring is a feature across the animal world and it doesn't go away once a baby is born ... or indeed when your children are fully grown! As my mother said to me after the birth of my first baby, once you have children, you become a hostage to fortune, never quite losing that need to know they are okay and happy.

Even where everything seems fine over the course of your pregnancy, you may find that you dwell on the 'what ifs' and there may be many times when the thought will come into your head that maybe something will happen or something will go wrong. There may be no obvious rationale for this heightened concern, other than 'Why *shouldn't* it happen to me?' For example, when I was pregnant for the third time, having already had two healthy children, I started to think that there might be something wrong with my baby simply because it might be 'my turn' – it wasn't and everything was completely normal but lots of people said to me afterwards, 'Oh, it's because it's your third baby', as if that alone explained it.

Sadly though, you may have a tangible reason for your fears because of a previously difficult pregnancy or birth, whether or not this led to a poor outcome. Your anxiety levels in these circumstances will naturally be higher and your confidence possibly lower because of your lived experience.

Whether you are just feeling anxious occasionally or it is an almost permanent state of mind, you may be able to reduce that anxiety by trying to ensure that you are making the safest choices for yourself and your baby. But then the question arises, what exactly does safety in childbirth mean? What does being safe feel like to you and is it the same for your family or your partner? We are all different: some may be extremely risk-averse in life generally, while others may be completely laid back and just deal with whatever comes when it happens, without spending too long worrying about it beforehand.

Wherever we are on the 'bell curve' of anxiety levels, we are receiving our maternity care within the context of today's medicalised model, in which the midwives and doctors who provide that care use a 'risk management' approach to safety, applying certain 'rules' to try to quantify, measure and control our individual risk. What this does, unfortunately, is focus attention on what might go wrong, so that the probability that everything will be alright has a tendency to get lost.

If your particular take on safety happens to align with this approach, you may be reassured by everything that is being offered to you. However, for others this viewpoint may feel completely unhelpful and do nothing to reassure them. The difficulty is that the system has evolved to try to 'process' everyone through the same journey in as efficient a manner as possible, whether or not it is relevant or desired; and, because the medical model's other feature is an increased fragmentation of care, the personal element of care is often lost. The woman as an individual may feel unsupported and lost in a system that simply doesn't have the capacity or structural framework to respond to her specific needs and anxieties, especially when these are emotional or psychological.

It is obvious of course that the pregnancy and childbirth journey does not operate in a vacuum separate from the rest of the developments in society. Globally there is a big increase in obesity rates, with diabetes and other serious health conditions reaching epidemic proportions. This in turn means a corresponding increase in the number of pregnancies in which a woman already has medical and health issues prior to becoming pregnant, so that, in order to have a safe pregnancy and birth, she will need close monitoring and may need regular treatment.

We need a system that is balanced. We need to pick up quickly and efficiently on genuine problems for an individual woman rather than applying tests and screening universally for all potential but still rare problems. As things stand at the moment, 99 per cent of women end up having a treatment or process done to them in order to find the 1 per cent who might have a particular condition.

There is a financial cost to this as well as an undermining of the normality of birth. We need to find a way of providing the information more sensitively so that women do not feel railroaded into having tests they are not comfortable with or are not likely to need. The woman-centred care described by the 1993 *Changing Childbirth: Report of the Expert Maternity Group*[4] (*see* page 221) may not have been fully realised yet, but there is a much better understanding today of the concept of informed choice and it is worth remembering that nothing should be done to you without your clear and expressed agreement.

If you don't understand what the test you are being offered is for, or what the benefits are compared to the risks, you have every right to ask as many questions as you need to reach an understanding of the options in order to make the choice that feels right for you.

Personal influences

Whatever the reasons are for you having picked up this book – you may just be curious, or you may already be seriously considering having your baby at home and are looking for some tips – the reality is that you probably will not know many others who have made the same choice or who are even considering it. This is mostly because having your baby in hospital is still currently the default option for the majority of women and most will give little thought to the possibility of doing it anywhere else. The other element that contributes to the low numbers of women who actively choose home birth is how it is viewed within the wider context of society.

There is an emotional and charged debate around having your baby at home that has little to do with facts but is nonetheless a powerful inhibitor when you start to weigh up the pros and cons for yourself. If you mention that you are considering having a home birth, the chances are you will have friends, acquaintances, colleagues and sometimes complete strangers keen to share their stories with you and give you the benefit of their experience, knowledge and sometimes dire warnings about the many – usually anecdotal – 'what ifs' and 'just-in-case' scenarios that they know of.

These stories may have the power to stop you in your tracks, introducing doubt and fear into your thinking, because everyone, from your parents, neighbours to sometimes your own GP, will have a personal, often negative, opinion about home birth that they often can't wait to pass on. Unfortunately, one result of this negativity is that, should there be a poor outcome at a home birth, the universal response tends to be 'If only you had been in hospital', with the implication that hospitals are always risk-free and that there are never any problems there.

Even if no one actually says it directly to the woman, she may think it herself or worry that this is how everyone will judge her. The decision about where to have your baby is therefore often framed as choosing between a place fraught with danger (your home) and one of safety (the hospital with its technology, equipment and medical expertise).

These negative stories and experiences are then amplified within the media, and sadly the public debate about issues of safety and risk in childbirth is often very superficial and polarised, which can be deeply unhelpful when you are weighing up your options and need balanced, accurate information on which to base your decision. There is usually little evidence of that in the emotionally charged and often dogmatic viewpoints expressed in the comment and opinion pieces that regularly fill the newspapers and where the facts and figures can be skewed either way – depending on the stance taken.

First-time mothers who opt for home birth face triple the risk of death or brain damage in child

Daily Mail (2011)[5]

This headline in the *Daily Mail* accompanied a report of the findings of the Birthplace in England study[6] in 2011. In fact, when examined a little more closely, it was disingenuous, to say the least, as the *Daily Mail* had compared the results for different groups of women and concluded that the risk of an adverse perinatal outcome for ALL women was 3.5 per 1,000 (i.e. 0.3 per cent) in a midwifery-led unit, but for women expecting their *first* baby it was 9.5 per 1,000 (or 0.9 per cent) at home. If one more accurately compared the results for all first-time babies across the different birth settings, the differences were less marked: midwifery-led unit 0.4 per cent; obstetric unit 0.5 per cent; home 0.9 per cent. So, although there is still a slightly increased risk of an adverse outcome for women having their first baby at home, it doesn't make for quite the same sensationalist headline. Nor, interestingly, did the *Daily Mail* include the fact that for women expecting a second or subsequent baby, the risk of an adverse outcome is actually slightly higher in an obstetric unit (0.3 per cent) than at home (0.2 per cent).

So does home birth deserve the bad press it often receives? If there is a common perception that it is an unsafe place to have your baby, why is that? It certainly doesn't fit with the facts or (as evidenced by the phenomenal global population growth of our species) the innate ability of reasonably fit and healthy women to give birth successfully and without medical intervention.

It is important to try to gain an understanding of where such antipathy to the idea of home birth comes from. Ultimately, to arrive at your own conclusions about what is the right decision for you (and your partner) regarding your chosen place of birth, you need to be able to make sense of the information that is available and test it against some objective measurements of the facts and figures. In Part 3 of this book I have revisited the findings of Marjorie Tew, a research statistician in the 1980s, whose analysis of the official data exposed the myth that hospital automatically means 'safe'.[7] I've also included a round-up of the latest evidence, all of which I hope will help you weigh up the risks and benefits for your particular circumstances.

Health reform and recent government policy

Building on the findings and conclusions of *Changing Childbirth* from the 1990s, health reform in this country over the past decade or so has been based on two key government policy documents: the *National Service Framework for Children, Young People and Maternity Services* (2004)[8] and *Maternity Matters* (2007).[9] The latter publication reconfirmed the importance of continuity and choice by setting out the 'four choices guarantee' – choice of how to access maternity care; choice of type of antenatal care; choice of place of birth; choice of place of postnatal care – for women, which was supposed to be fully implemented by 2009.

Here we are in 2016, however, with no discernible difference as yet to the percentage of women who are now able to access a reliable home birth service in their area. You would be forgiven for wondering what it will take to make continuity of carer and choice of home birth a realistic and attainable option for any woman wanting to access it in the 21st century.

One part of the answer might lie with the publication, in December 2014, of new national guidelines. I have copied out the most relevant parts of these in Part 3 of this book (*see* page 245) because, if you request a home birth and have any problems, you could quote from them to support your case.

In a nutshell, the new guidance recommends a much more proactive policy of increasing the provision of home birth services to support those women who wish to have their baby at home. It also underlines the need for women considering the place of birth to be provided with more detailed information about the risk of transfer and the risk of obstetric intervention across all the different settings.

This is key because now the most up-to-date evidence available, from the Birthplace in England Programme,[10] underpins, confirms and strengthens the conclusions Marjorie Tew arrived at almost 30 years ago: namely that giving birth in an obstetric unit, when you are a healthy woman with a well-grown, healthy baby on board – most women, according to the National Institute for Health and Care Excellence (NICE[11]) – is not necessarily any safer for you and your baby, and should, in fact, be avoided if you would prefer not to have unnecessary interventions and want the best outcome for you and your baby.[12] 'Back to the future' is a phrase that springs to mind.

The other potential game changer is the National Maternity Review, entitled 'Better Births: Improving outcomes of maternity services in England'[13] that has been published as this book goes to print in February 2016. It was tasked by NHS England to gather evidence about best practice, both in this country and abroad, as well as the views of many stakeholders from across England – service users from a wide range of backgrounds, providers, healthcare professionals, politicians, managers, commissioners etc. The review team wanted to understand what the shortcomings of the current service are, what each individual's own experiences have been – either as users or providers – and what contributors thought were the most important issues to be addressed.

As a member of that review panel, I was privileged to work alongside many dedicated and knowledgeable professionals and what we heard from around the country left us in no doubt that there is widespread and unanimous agreement about the need for more continuity of care, as well as much more effective policies to encourage more women to have their baby away from an obstetric unit.

We spent many months debating the issues and working through different ideas and proposals and the result is, I believe, an inspired vision for a modern maternity service. If the recommendations are implemented, they will deliver safer, more personalised and kinder care for all women and every baby, improve outcomes and reduce inequalities. In order to do this, the review identifies seven key priorities, all focused on how to bring about some of the cultural and operational changes that are needed for wholesale system reform.

The challenge, in today's climate of austerity, is how to provide all this within the existing financial and workforce constraints. The report has included costings and considerations whose conclusions are that, rather than asking for additional resources, it is more about reorganising those we already have (especially midwives) to work in very different ways. There are also savings to be made, for example if there are fewer interventions and more normal births outside of obstetric units.

The report is well worth a read, especially as there is a proposal for a small number of interested Clinical Commissioning Groups (CCGs) to pilot a personal maternity budget scheme, where a woman will be able to access e-vouchers to pay the provider of her choice directly. It is envisaged that this will act as a lever for change by giving women more say in where they want to have their baby and who can look after them. If you are interested you can ask if your CCG is taking part.

Thinking Ahead

Although there will be times when you will feel as if you have been pregnant for an eternity and wish the whole thing didn't take so long, one of the useful things about pregnancy lasting for around 40 weeks is that you've got lots of time to think about, research and put into practice all the different ingredients that will help make your home birth more likely to be successful. It is important to really think about what is important to you. Use the time wisely and try not to leave everything to the last minute, especially since some things will be best achieved by embarking on them early on in the pregnancy – for example, making healthy choices about what you're eating.

Optimal nutrition

Eating well for a healthy baby is something that many women focus on. What you choose to put into your body when you are pregnant has important repercussions and it's a great time to stop and reflect about what constitutes a good diet and introduce some changes to your eating habits if they are needed! When I was first pregnant with my eldest, Lucy, I became hyper-aware of everything I was eating and I realised very quickly that my overall diet could do with some revising – years of working late and then going straight to the pub, and snacking on packets of crisps or a piece of toast late at night had created some bad habits. Although meeting Peter, my husband, had improved these considerably – he was much more health conscious than me – becoming pregnant was the springboard to a permanent change in my behaviour.

I bought *The Food Scandal* by Caroline Walker when it was published in 1985 and it was a Eureka moment for me. The provenance and preparation of food was definitely something I became much more interested in and aware of during my first pregnancy and it then helped to inform my thoughts about breastfeeding and weaning further down the line. Finding out you are expecting a baby will often be the catalyst for introducing all sorts of changes in your life. These could be ones you have been contemplating for some time, but it may be the dawning realisation that you are responsible for another human being that finally propels you to act.

In the early weeks you may feel really nauseous and be limited in what you can keep down. You may only feel like eating very bland, carb-heavy food, but once you start to feel a little better it's really good to think in more detail about what kinds of food are better for you and what will help grow a healthy baby. At Neighbourhood Midwives we have a simple handout we share with all our clients, which has some basic principles about nutrition, but nothing is set in stone and your own choices will depend on your particular situation and culture.

As a general rule, avoid processed foods and, if possible, reduce wheat – it is one of the most common food intolerances and often causes bloating and fluid retention – and increase protein intake. There is lots of information available about good nutrition in pregnancy and also what foods to avoid. The main point is don't leave making these changes until the last week of pregnancy!

Top tips for healthy eating

The nutritional advice of Neighbourhood Midwives is based on a well-balanced, low-GI diet and is appropriate for all pregnant women. It may be particularly useful for women who are already overweight, have a history of large weight gain in pregnancy or a history of large babies.

As a general rule, cook with basic fresh foods, and avoid ready-meals and processed foods wherever possible. Make sure you include the following:

- **Plenty of protein:** Good sources of protein are meat, soy products, mycoprotein, dairy, eggs, beans and pulses. Eat five helpings daily if a meat eater, seven if vegetarian and nine if vegan.
- **Complex carbohydrates:** These include beans, pulses and high-fibre wholegrain foods such as wholemeal bread, brown rice, wholegrain pasta. Try to eat complex carbohydrates with a protein rather than on their own, and only one portion of wholemeal bread (two slices) each day. *Reduce* the amount of simple carbohydrates (e.g. white bread, rice, pasta).
- **Plenty of Vitamin B (complex):** Found in wholegrains, meat and nuts.
- **Plenty of Vitamin C:** Found in fresh fruit and vegetables.
- **Plenty of water:** Tap or bottled is fine.
- **Salt to taste:** A good sea or mineral salt is best.

For all women, but particularly for those who have had large babies (over 4kg) or have had problems with blood sugar control, we advise:

- **Don't eat too much fruit:** You should eat more veg than fruit every day and avoid fresh fruit juices altogether.
- **No 'empty calories':** Avoid things like white bread, cakes, biscuits, crisps and fizzy drinks.
- **Reduce the amount of saturated fat:** Avoid fatty meat, too much butter, pastries, cakes, biscuits etc.
- **Exercise regularly:** Take a brisk walk or go for a swim.

Decision-making in pregnancy

If we are feeling unwell and need to make contact with our GP or other healthcare professionals, we tend to put ourselves in their hands as we're looking for a diagnosis or remedy and we rely to a large extent on the fact that they hold the specialist knowledge and can give us the treatment we need to get better.

Although things have changed in recent years with increased access to information via the Internet, the GP's surgery is still usually our first port of call if we feel ill enough and, from the healthcare professionals' point of view, their job is to try to work out what is wrong with us and then treat/refer us accordingly.

Having a baby, however, is one of those life events that doesn't fit neatly into this pattern. Getting pregnant and growing a baby isn't an illness, it doesn't require a diagnosis from a specialist, and most women, once they know they are pregnant, instinctively know what's right for them. Healthcare professionals, especially midwives, are there to support and advise women in their decision-making process but not to take it over or dictate what anyone should or shouldn't be doing. Unfortunately though, for any number of reasons, the journey through our maternity services for many women is now a series of short 10–15-minute appointments where you will be given lots of information, often via leaflets, sometimes by the same person but more often, especially in London, by someone different every time.

The process is generally unsatisfactory for both women and midwives, with a lot of bureaucratic 'box ticking' and form filling and not enough time to have a proper discussion about any of the choices, concerns or ideas about different aspects of the pregnancy that individuals might be mulling over. In this scenario, it can often come down to the midwife steering a woman in a certain direction, one that is in line with the hospital's protocols and guidelines. It may be that you would have arrived at that conclusion yourself anyway, but nevertheless, it is questionable whether the process and end result are genuinely informed decision-making and consent.

This may or may not be important to you, but even if you are happy to accept the various procedures and processes you are being booked in for, it is still important that you properly understand their purpose and, if you don't, that you feel able to ask questions to get some clarity before agreeing. There have been situations where a woman was not given the whole picture and this had ramifications for her that were not always positive. A recent Supreme Court ruling in Scotland about such a case has made it crystal clear that every woman has a right to informed consent and that healthcare professionals, however busy or rushed they are, must, by law, ensure that the woman understands the balance of risks of any treatment she is being offered.[14]

This lack of proper discussion is regrettable because, unless you are very determined, it can begin to feel as though you are just on a conveyor belt, with lots of things being arranged for you, without the need for much engagement on your part. Personally, as a midwife, I think it's much more satisfactory when a woman says, 'I've thought about this deeply, I've read around the subject/ looked at the evidence and this is my decision, based on what I know I want for myself and for my baby.' Being able to make a properly informed decision for yourself means that then you will own it and take personal responsibility for it, which in turn is all part of becoming a mother and feeling empowered to make the right decisions for you and your family. Feeling as if you have to agree to something simply because that is what happens at the hospital you are booked into is simply not acceptable.

Taking responsibility for the decisions you make – and understanding the pros and cons of a particular choice for you as an individual is especially important when it comes to considering where to have your baby, because, of all the decisions you make during pregnancy, it is likely to be the one that, if/when you tell them, friends, family, peers, work colleagues and even passing acquaintances will often feel they can question and ask, sometimes incredulously, 'Are you sure?', 'What if something terrible happens?', 'What if something goes wrong?' We explore this issue elsewhere, but if you wish to plan a home birth, chances are you will be thinking about it yourself anyway – not many women end up with a home birth without some degree of self-determination!

Choosing your caregiver

Once you have confirmed your pregnancy, the next step is to decide where to book in for your midwifery/obstetric care. If you have found out very early, and with the pregnancy tests that are around now, that is increasingly common, you don't need to rush to choose; and even once you have booked somewhere, you can change your mind at any point should you want to.

You may have been very clear from before you were pregnant that you want to have your baby at home, but equally it may not have occurred to you until something changed your mind or the seed was planted by a chance remark, possibly quite late in pregnancy. Either way, one of the things you should really consider is who is going to be with you on this journey into motherhood? If planning a home birth, who are you going to invite into your home and how can you ensure you feel comfortable with them, trust them and feel safe enough to put yourself and your baby in their hands?

One of the problems in our current system is that, even if you have a reasonably reliable home birth service in your area, you may have no idea who will actually turn up on the day/ night and what, if anything, can be done if it is someone you don't feel comfortable with. The answer to this, by the way, is that you can request another midwife, but in reality that is very hard to do and there may not be anyone else available.

The best service, in my opinion, and the one that evidence suggests has the best outcomes and satisfaction scores,[15] is one in which you meet one or two midwives at the start of your pregnancy whom you get to know really well and who will come to you when you start your labour, be there for the duration of the birth and then provide your postnatal care too.

This type of service is known as 'caseloading': one midwife looks after a specific group of women, often in partnership with a 'buddy' and with support from a small team. It describes a way of providing care that puts the relationship between the woman and the midwife at the centre and is somewhat at odds with the large, bureaucratic and fragmented service that is currently the norm, where midwives are more commonly organised to work in ways that suit the system rather than the individuals.

Caseloading is known as the 'gold standard' of care. Along with many changes now appearing in maternity services, the interest in and opportunities for caseload midwifery are re-emerging, helped perhaps by TV dramas such as *Call the Midwife*, which celebrates the relationships between the local midwives portrayed in the series and the women in their care.

If you do some local research and find that there is a caseload team (where each midwife looks after her own 'caseload' of women) in your area, see if you can book in with them. Alternatively, there are some areas that have a dedicated home birth team, so, if you have already decided that is what you want, get in touch sooner rather than later in case they have a cap on numbers.

The beauty of a caseloading service is that it gives you the time to build a relationship with your midwife, and, if you aren't 100 per cent sure about where you want to have your baby, you don't have to make a definite decision about the place of birth at the beginning of your care. You can talk it through with her over the course of your pregnancy and even leave it until the labour itself (i.e. when you start having contractions, your caseload midwife will usually come and assess you at home, at which point you can discuss how you feel, decide how the labour is going and decide which option feels most comfortable).

Where these sorts of services exist, the home birth rate tends to show a sharp rise as women can (and do!) choose that option very late in the day. The first birth I saw, when I was thinking about becoming a midwife, was of my youngest sister's third baby, now a tall young man in his twenties. My sister had a community midwife visit her at home when she was in early labour (she was receiving her midwifery care through the DOMINO scheme, which has largely disappeared now, although a description of it can be found at www.eumom.ie/pregnancy/the-domino-scheme-explained). When she realised she was doing rather well and was enjoying being in her own bath, she asked if she could just stay at home to have the baby rather than transfer to hospital, to which the answer was, 'Yes, of course.' Within a very short time another midwife arrived for the second stage of labour and I was privileged to witness a wonderful home birth, which pretty much sealed my decision that this was what I wanted to do!

If there are none of these options available in your area, it is time to start asking why not, given that the national guidelines are now actively promoting 'out of hospital' birth, which obviously includes home birth. The National Maternity Review report, published in February 2016 and discussed on page 21, has proposed the setting up of 'community hubs', based much closer to women's homes and with a wide range of services available from them, including midwifery and obstetric care, peer support groups, and independent midwifery practices, accredited to provide NHS care. You could ask if your local CCG is planning to develop one near you.

As well as thinking about your hospital or midwifery provider, there are other options you can consider. Doulas, for example, are an increasingly popular choice, especially in those areas where there is a particular problem such as a shortage of midwives or chronic lack of continuity (London being an example). A doula is usually an experienced woman who can provide emotional and practical support to you and your partner, before, during and after childbirth. She will not be able to provide any clinical care but may well offer some complementary therapies as part of her 'package'. She may have had a baby before, but not necessarily. You can easily research who is in your area (http://doula.org.uk/content/what-doula) and arrange to meet them during pregnancy to decide if they are the right person for you.

Antenatal education

Another important element to think about in pregnancy is booking yourself into some antenatal classes. There is a plethora of different organisations that offer them in a variety of formats. The National Childbirth Trust (NCT) is perhaps the most well known of the private options but there are many other providers. The NHS often has local classes as well. It's a question of researching what's in your area and choosing one that feels the best fit for you (I suggest you do this relatively early as sometimes these classes get booked up very quickly).

It isn't just about information gathering though; it's also about meeting up regularly with a group of women, with and without their partners, probably all reasonably local to you, who are expecting their baby around the same sort of time. The connection that you can make with other women who are experiencing the same life event as yourself will often lead to the development of lifelong friendships – for example, I am still in touch with some members of my first NCT group from 30 years ago – but even if it doesn't, sharing the same or similar anxieties and concerns is a key element of learning and absorption of information. You can bat ideas around between each other and it's such a helpful way of thinking through all the different elements of this journey you are on and what is really important to you along the way.

How much research, information gathering and preparation should you do? There are some very different schools of thought about this. Who you are as a person, what you do for a living, what your memories and childhood experiences have been etc. will all play a part in your personal approach to preparing for childbirth. Some women feel that giving birth is a natural, instinctive thing and that you'll just confuse things if you do too much research – in other words, you can over-think it and it's better just to get on with living life day to day, with the pregnancy almost in the background, and then at the birth what will be will be. For others, it might be an opportunity to really try to understand what is happening inside your body, why you are experiencing these unusual or different, sometimes unpleasant, sensations and what will happen during labour and birth. Sometimes, particularly if you are someone used to being fully in control of your life, the slightly 'out-of-control' feelings pregnancy can engender cause anxiety and stress, and overarching all of this is the generally increased level of fear that is much more present today than it ever used to be. I explore the 'fear factor' more when looking at risk (*see* page 228), but it has played its part in the rise of hypnobirthing, hypnotherapy and mindfulness as methods of managing the feelings of anxiety and sometimes panic that increasingly seem to accompany thoughts of labour and birth in pregnancy.

The approach and attitude you adopt during pregnancy will depend on who you are and there are absolutely no hard-and-fast rules – it's about what works for you. However, if you are thinking about having a home birth, or home birth is suggested to you as an option, it's a good idea to have at least thought through what that might entail and to have given yourself some time to consider the pros and cons for you in your particular situation. It can be rather overwhelming just randomly surfing the Internet – there is an enormous amount of information out there and some sort of structure or connection is very helpful, especially hearing questions or the thoughts of other women in your antenatal group that may not have occurred to you.

Networking in pregnancy

I've already touched on this in the antenatal education section, but I can't emphasise enough the importance of building networks, as part of your general preparation during pregnancy, for after your baby is born. It's such a good way of minimising the risk of becoming isolated during the postnatal period (we really are not very good in Western society at supporting vulnerable new mothers to manage their lives with their babies), but it does need to be actively thought about and planned.

Join as many classes as you want. Antenatal education classes, yoga, hypnobirthing and home birth groups are all widely available, particularly in large cities, and provide an opportunity to meet pregnant women who will be just as keen to meet others in the same situation. Try to get to know the members of your new 'group' during pregnancy to the point where you feel comfortable making regular contact with them post-baby – it might seem too daunting to start forging new relationships while sleep-deprived and perhaps feeling vulnerable and unsure of yourself.

As mammals, we are naturally social animals who function best in social groups. If you look at how traditional communities operate, the women will often work together and share tasks, including childrearing. The way in which we organise ourselves in today's 'modern' society is in sharp contrast to this model. Our nuclear family, often living many miles or even continents away from other family members, does not provide the opportunity to share the burden of household tasks and childcare with others. Women can end up alone with their small baby for many hours in the day once the initial support of the first couple of weeks has ended and their partners have returned to work. Remaining in isolation behind your front door and feeling lonely can increase the risk of postnatal depression and low self-confidence.

You may be leaving a busy, lively and sociable office to go on maternity leave, and therefore miss the stimulation of work and the company of others. I'm not suggesting that in the first couple of weeks after your baby is born you go around madly socialising – quite the opposite, as we'll discuss elsewhere. However, once you are into your third week – by which time, one hopes, you are beginning to recover from the birth and are getting more familiar with feeding and caring for your baby – now is the time to make sure you are able to get plenty of support through a variety of means. By interacting with other women (both older and younger), including family, friends, role models and peers, you can enjoy your time with your baby while getting out and about. If you put some time and effort into developing those relationships and building your networks while you are pregnant, it will pay dividends after your baby is born. You will have a choice of friends to call and meet up with, and you and your baby are likely to be much happier if you are a socially active mum.

Getting Things Ready

Neighbourhood Midwives always provide women with suggestions of things to collect together ready for the big day. I have included our checklist below and will go into more detail a little later under 'Other provisions'. Of course, you can add anything you like to the list! It may be helpful to put everything into a couple of boxes marked 'Mum' and 'Baby', so that items are easily identifiable and accessible and you're not having to give directions about where to find things when you should be switching off and focusing on labour. Ideally, aim to have everything organised by about 37 weeks.

Your home birth checklist

The setting for labour and birth:

- Space (just a little) to move around, squat, lean and kneel in.
- Lighting, music and candles to create a calm atmosphere for you during labour.
- Temperature control. While you are in labour you may want the room temperature to be as cool as if you were exercising. However, the baby needs to be born into a warm room (at least 20°C), so it's helpful to have a

quick way of heating the room if it is spring or autumn or if your central heating takes a while to warm up (e.g. fan heater/oil-filled radiator).

- Plenty of pillows/cushions/old duvets etc.
- Something waterproof to protect the carpet, sofa or bed (e.g. a cheap shower curtain as they have a non-slip surface or dust sheets from a DIY shop).
- Any old sheets or linen (e.g. fitted sheets and/or old double duvet cover – prospective grandparents are often a useful supplier!)
- Disposable bed mats or changing mats (available from large chemists and babycare shops).
- Two clean tea trays to put equipment on (and tea towels to cover).
- Torch and batteries.

Food and drink:

- Light nutritious snacks (e.g. fruit juice, yogurt, bananas, nuts and seeds, snack bars, toast, honey).
- Nourishing fluids of choice.
- Bendy straws – it is easier to drink from a glass with a bendy straw when in strong labour, particularly if you are on all fours.
- Snacks and drinks for the midwives!!

Other supplies:

- Hot water bottle or wheat bag to put on your back or bump in labour, or to warm towels or clothes for the baby.

- Camera.
- Plenty of hot water and towels for showers and baths during labour and afterwards.
- Kitchen and toilet rolls.
- Antiseptic spray and/or wipes.
- Roll of cotton wool and nappies for baby.
- Baby wipes for general use.
- Box of large tissues.
- Strong black refuse sacks.
- Comfortable clothes to wear in labour –baggy, soft old T-shirts are ideal.
- Two or three, preferably new, flannels for cooling hot face or for hot compresses on the perineum if necessary or desired.
- Plastic bowl (for hot water compresses or if you are sick).
- Empty, clean 1-litre ice cream container for the placenta (if you wish to keep it).
- Big, old towels and at least four or five small old towels for the baby.
- Old towelling dressing gown – great for when you get out of the pool, to stop you getting cold.
- Larger size than usual knickers to wear with pads after birth.
- Maternity pads (large sanitary pads), preferably ones without a plastic backing.
- Warm clothes to dress baby in and two knitted baby hats to prevent baby getting cold.
- Nappies.
- Celebratory food and drink for toasting the baby.

- Nice 'staying-in-bed clothes' to encourage lying back
  and enjoying a rest for a few days after the birth. A nice
  dressing gown for entertaining but not doing any work in!
- A freezer full of easy-to-prepare meals or a partner who
  can prepare nutritious food.
- A bag packed for hospital in case the need arises,
  containing nightclothes, toiletries, knickers and pads,
  baby clothes and nappies.

The pool (if you are using one):

- Plenty of hot water (check your hot water system and
  know how to keep it on constantly).
- Universal tap adaptor for filling the pool.
- Sieve to keep pool clear.
- New hose pipe for filling the pool.
- Bucket for topping up the pool with hot water.

The midwife will bring her own supplies, of course, some of which she may leave with you a couple of weeks before the birth. If she does, add them to your own pile and then you know you've got everything you need ready in one place for when the baby decides to come.

Physical and psychological preparation

Labour has often been likened to running a marathon and there are certainly a lot of similarities: pacing yourself, making sure that you're taking in enough fluids to stay well hydrated, not exhausting yourself by starting too fast at the beginning and then running out of steam half way through. All of those things can directly relate to labour, which, particularly for a first-time baby but even with second or subsequent ones, tends to be a challenging physical exertion. So the fitter and more mentally prepared you are, the better you will be at coping with it.

It's not an absolute guarantee of course, because medical conditions or complicating factors can arise whether you're fit or not, but being physically fit certainly won't do any harm and it's useful to build psychological resilience and prepare yourself for the challenge. My personal take on the process of labour is that nature has intentionally made it rather hard work as a preparation for parenthood, which is the real challenge you're being prepared for. Childbirth is a rite of passage and if you have a positive birth experience, it can lay down a really good foundation for all those challenges ahead, providing a great start to your parenting journey.

As with any of the challenges we take on in life, it can really help to consciously take personal responsibility to prepare yourself well, and part of that preparation is to think about developing strategies to manage the ups and downs of labour. Going back to the analogy of the marathon, the more training and preparation you put in, generally the better able you are to cope with those low points – for example, when you think that it's never going to end or that you just can't do it any more, and the difficult transitional phases, when you might lose the plot for a while and feel lost in the enormity of it all.

The challenge and reward is to push through those periods and to get to that moment of birth ... when you hold your baby in your arms, when the sheer hard slog of the previous hours is over and can be almost immediately forgotten because at that moment mostly what you feel is enormous relief, triumph and elation. To reach that point, you may have had to dig deep into the core of your being to find the strength and inner resilience to meet that challenge – hence the elation and sense of achievement when it has ended.

I often wonder why it is that we reward people (usually men) for doing the most random things – walking across the globe for instance, climbing mountains, or going on a 1,000-mile bike ride. We applaud and congratulate those individuals who do such things to challenge themselves, yet every woman in labour is being tested and challenged – and for a much more significant purpose. But for some reason we don't view their challenge in the same way, we doubt their ability to give birth without help and offer to rescue them from the process either with drugs or with other interventions to help. We celebrate the arrival of a new little person but not women's ability to rise to the challenge of an unmedicated labour with the sense of empowerment it can bring.

This is not about judging anyone for the choices they make – far from it – it is just an observation that managing labour without intervention is often derided by some in the media as a pointless choice, like refusing to have pain relief for a trip to the dentist (and my guess is that anyone who compares labour to a toothache has never had a baby). It is curious to me as to why that should be.

There are lots of different ways to prepare physically: yoga, hypnobirthing and sophrology, to name a few. We'll talk about these in more detail in the section on pain relief in labour, but they are really good ways of preparing your body *and* your mind.

Thinking about the physical preparation in a more holistic way is key to increasing the likelihood of success. There are tools to help you as well. The Epi-No® is one of my favourites – it is a muscle exercising and stretching device for the pelvic floor and perineum. As well as the physical preparation it provides, I think it also helps you to connect emotionally and psychologically with that part of your body again. It can also familiarise you with the sensations of stretching, so that as the baby comes down the birth canal in the second stage of labour you are less likely to instinctively contract those muscles in response. Have a look at the Epi-No website for more information about how it works (www.epi-no.co.uk) or, if you don't fancy that or can't afford it, perineal massage is the other option. There are lots of different descriptions around – for example, have a look in the pregnancy portal on our Neighbourhood Midwives website (www.neighbourhoodmidwives.org.uk/pregnancy-portal/pregnancy).

Finally, get into the habit, once you have started to feel your baby move, of tuning in to his or her movements throughout the day. Although all babies will have short episodes of sleep, these will normally only last between 20 and 40 minutes and never longer than 90 minutes. Each baby is individual so there is no average or set number of kicks to monitor. More importantly, it is about tuning into your own baby's pattern of movement and contacting your midwife if you are concerned that they are less frequent or have changed from their usual pattern. Check out this website for more details: www.countthekicks.org.uk.

The birth environment

This is the fun part of planning your home birth. You don't have to worry that the place you will be giving birth in will feel alien to you or that you won't know until you get there whether or not the room with a birthpool is available, or whether the midwife-led birth centre is closed because of staff shortages. You can decide what feels right for you because you are in control of all these elements and, since it is your home, everything will feel very familiar and safe.

All you have to do is decide where in your home you think you want to give birth. Sometimes women know instinctively that they want to be in a certain room, a certain space – it could be your bedroom, the bathroom or perhaps the kitchen – and you can always change your mind on the day. If you are planning to give birth in a pool, however, you'll need to consider where to put that up as once it's full of water you won't be moving it anywhere!

Once you are in active labour, you might want to tuck yourself away in a quiet corner and stay there. If there are other people in the house, this might be more important than if you have the whole place to yourself; but either way, you'll need easy access to the loo and enough space to move around in, things to lean against and places where you can kneel, squat and lie down.

Alternatively, you might find that you want to move around from room to room – for example, you might go into the bathroom or shower, or down to the kitchen for something to eat. You might even use the stairs to get contractions going again if they slow down or to help get the baby into a better position – this might be at the suggestion of your midwife, but the important thing is that it's still your choice. Lots of women like to move around more in early labour but tend to settle into a particular space as labour progresses. I remember being downstairs in my kitchen when in early labour with my second baby, being quite sociable with Patti, my mother-in-law who lived with us, and a couple of friends who had popped in, plus my daughter Lucy and Peter; but at some point something changed and, as the contractions picked up in intensity and I had to give them more attention, I needed to get away from everyone, to find my quiet space (for me it was my bedroom) so that I could begin to focus and go into myself more.

Like every aspect of labour, though, this is very individual and I've been at births where the more the merrier is the order of the day, with the labouring woman drawing strength and energy from those around her.

When thinking about the environment where you plan to give birth, you can create a very calm atmosphere, which enhances your own sense of relaxation and supports your being in 'the zone', using cushions, music, candles – all these are elements to think about and getting them ready is a lovely part of the nesting and preparation that most women want to do, usually driven very strongly by their hormones!

Putting together your own musical playlist is so easy to do these days and could be anything from whale sounds to heavy rock, although it might be worth overseeing anything your partner puts together as you don't want to be taken by surprise by his choice of 'upbeat' music belting out in the middle of a particularly intense contraction!

Most women will opt for dim lighting if given the choice. Candles can be the perfect way to achieve this, especially those with your favourite essential oil ... or check out some of the most appropriate to enhance your mood and sense of release and relaxation. If you are labouring in the daytime you might want to have the option of darkening the room with temporary covers for the windows.

Temperature-wise, much depends on the time of year. If it's summer and very warm, you'll want to have things to cool you down, such as a fan or even air-conditioning (you can hire mobile units if there is the risk of a heatwave). Equally, if it's winter and the middle of a cold snap, you'll want to be warm enough to feel comfortable.

Whatever the weather, being in labour is usually the equivalent of a pretty vigorous workout and so you'll want to be able to cool down if you tend to overheat in such circumstances. Flannels, which can be rinsed in cold water for your face and neck, work well, as does a fine mist spray.

Depending on the time of year, it is also worth thinking about a quick way to heat the room in preparation for when your baby is about to be born, especially if you are not in warm water. Closing windows to prevent direct draughts or having some sort of convector heater handy would be useful if your central heating takes a while to come on or you don't want/ need to heat the whole house. The baby has been used to your body temperature of around 37°C for the past nine months and so ideally, if they come out into a reasonably warm environment initially, they won't cool too quickly; then having them skin to skin will help them to stay nice and warm and will help them to regulate their core temperature.

Other provisions:

- **Birth pool:** If you're planning a water birth and you want to buy a birthing pool, the easiest way is to research well ahead of time and see which one most appeals, either because of cost or ease of use. There are a few other things to think about: usually when you buy an inflatable pool you will be sent an additional liner, but check that this is the case and what else is included in the price before you purchase it. If you do a trial run and use a liner, make sure you have an unused one ready for the birth itself. You will also need a hose pipe, and tap connector. Make sure the hose pipe reaches the preferred position for your pool and that the connector fits your particular tap. It's also good to have a sieve to keep the pool clear and a water thermometer to monitor the temperature, which is recommended as being 35–37°C, although recent evidence suggests the optimal temperature should be guided by maternal comfort. Have a bucket handy so that you can take cool water out prior to topping up with hot as necessary.

- **Nest building:** If you have, or can borrow, lots of pillows, cushions, a spare duvet or two and maybe a beanbag, you can build an early labour nest on your bed. The idea is that you create a big pile of all these items that you can lean against on your mattress. This prevents your knees from getting sore and you can relax into the nest in-between those early contractions, which are just a bit too much to manage lying down but aren't quite established enough to be classed as active labour. It's important to conserve energy at this stage by using the gaps between contractions to snooze or doze before the next one starts. You will be surprised how easy it is to drift off, even if the contractions feel quite close together, especially if you don't have to keep shifting position but can kneel upright to breathe through them and then just sink back into your nest each time they ebb away.

- **Waterproof sheet:** You'll need to have something waterproof to protect your carpet, settee, chairs, bed, mattress, duvet etc. You can buy one in any DIY store. It's worth spending a little more to get a cotton or hessian polythene-backed one that drapes easily, is not too slippy and is a little more robust than thin ones that may tear – you really don't want to have to deal with stains on your carpet after the birth!

- **Old sheets and towels:** On top of your waterproof sheet it's worth gathering together some old sheets or old duvet covers that can act as another layer and also cover sofas, cushions, beds etc. Try to collect lots of old towels as well, particularly if you're planning a water birth (you can never have too many towels!). You'll need different sizes, including small ones to dry the baby, who will come out wet and therefore cool quickly, and some bigger ones for you, particularly if you're getting in and out of the pool.

- **Disposable waterproof mats:** Often the midwives will bring these, but it's worth getting a couple of packs from a chemist or supermarket. They can be put down over the old sheets where you are kneeling and then replaced as necessary, wrapped and thrown away. You can also use them on your bed for the first couple of days once you've had your baby and they are handy for changing the baby on the bed in front of you if you don't have immediate access to a more substantial changing mat.

- **Tea trays:** This suggestion is one of my personal favourites, which I have used for years. It's a simple but effective way of ensuring you are not restricted to staying in one place to give birth, (i.e. next to where the midwife has set up her 'resuscitation station'). I lay my equipment out on each of the trays, one for the woman with all the relevant supplies in readiness, including oxytocic drugs for the third stage (delivery of the placenta) and one for the baby with resuscitation equipment, cord clamp etc. If, for whatever reason, you then decide you want or need to move somewhere else for the birth, then I simply pick up the tea tray and follow you into the bathroom or wherever else in the house you end up. Along with the tea trays we ask for a couple of clean tea towels, which we use to cover everything prior to use. The more things we can use that belong to you, rather than bringing things in, the better it is from an infection point of view.

- **Torch and batteries:** These are always handy to have just in case there is a power cut at the crucial moment. Although midwives generally carry their own, there is no harm in having a back-up.

- **Food and drink:** Thinking ahead of time, you could start getting a few snacks together to maintain or restore your energy levels during labour. Some will have a longer sell-by date than others so add things at the last minute as appropriate. Glucose sweets, cereal bars, raisins and other dried fruits and seeds can all be bought well ahead of time, while you just need to keep supplies of light, nutritious snacks such as fruit juice, yogurt, bananas, honey and bread for toast topped up. I recommend making up some ice cubes of frozen juice – orange and apple work well – so you can crunch on them during labour and in-between contractions. They are very refreshing and will give you a quick energy hit. Also, don't forget to think about food and drink for after the birth This might be your favourite meal and a bottle of champagne, or perhaps a mug of tea and hot, buttered toast! It is also really worth using the nesting period leading up to the labour to stock your freezer full of pre-cooked meals that your partner can easily get out and defrost in those first few days after your baby arrives, when cooking and preparing meals will be the last thing on anyone's mind. Finally, don't forget that we midwives really appreciate some snacks and drinks being available too!

- **Bendy straws:** A must! It's not easy to tip your head back to drink from a glass or bottle if you're in the pool, for example, or kneeling over. But someone just gently putting a drink in front of you with a bendy straw means that you're not having to disrupt your concentration or your position – you can easily take a quick sip without having to move at all.

- **Hot water bottle, heating pad or wheat pack:** Often localised warmth can be very effective at easing discomfort if you are suffering from backache (either generalised or because of the baby's position). You can also use warmth in the first few days after the baby is born to help ease any afterpains in your womb, which can feel like quite strong contractions the more babies you have had.

- **Camera:** Nowadays, with most people using smart phones, it's unlikely you won't have something close by to capture those first moments or to record your journey through labour. That's another conversation to be had: whether you'd like photos of the actual birth and, if so, who will take responsibility for taking them.

- **Flannels:** Two or three clean new flannels are useful, both for cooling you down, as previously mentioned, and for the midwife to use as a hot perineal compress as the baby is stretching you just before birth – it can feel wonderful!

- **Clothes for you:** If you want to, you can think about what clothes you might want to wear, at least in the earlier stages of labour, and put them to one side so that they aren't in the wash and unavailable when you go into labour. You may well end up wearing nothing, of course, especially if you plan to use a pool, but comfortable, baggy old clothes are ideal for pottering about in during the early stages. An old dressing gown is good too – something you can easily slip on and off when you're getting in and out of the pool for any reason, to stop you getting cold. Also, think about buying some new extra large pants for after you've had your baby – you probably won't want to go straight back to wearing thongs and anyway, they aren't very good at keeping sanitary pads in place. In the early days you'll need maternity pads (available from most pharmacies and large supermarkets), not the thinner ones with plastic backing. Not only are the latter not absorbent enough, but the plastic backing doesn't allow air to circulate – important if you have a tear or episiotomy that needs to heal. For the first few days following the birth, staying in pyjamas or leggings and T-shirt will, one hopes, remind you that you should be upstairs resting (more on this later) and will be easy for breastfeeding. Nursing bras can also be bought in advance.

Bra fitting services are available in lots of shops or you can measure yourself to estimate what size you will need.

- **Clothes for your baby:** You can keep this very simple: a vest, babygro (an all-in-one sleepsuit) and maybe a hat is all you will need, plus a cardigan and shawl or blanket if your baby is born during colder temperatures. You will also need nappies, of course, which I suggest are disposable in the first instance. Even if you plan to use the washable, reusable ones, you might want to save them for a little later as trying to work out how to put them on while seriously sleep-deprived might be a challenge too far in the early days!

- **Hospital bag:** This is worth packing in advance so that, should you need or want to transfer to an obstetric unit during labour, you don't have to think about what to pack. You'll only require a few things: clothes to come home in, toiletries, maternity pads, clean knickers (or disposable ones), some baby clothes and nappies.

Planning for the day

The Birth Talk

This is a regular part of our service at Neighbourhood Midwives, and most other midwifery providers will offer something very similar. Towards the end of pregnancy – at around 36 or 37 weeks – we schedule in a longer session, ideally in the evening so that you and your birth partner can both be involved. It's an opportunity to recap on everything that has been discussed during the pregnancy so far, as well as talking through how labour might start and ensuring you know who to contact and how. The areas we cover include:

- **Practical planning:**
  This covers all the practical aspects of being ready and organised on the day. Go through the list of things to prepare and check with your midwife what she'll be bringing and what you need to provide. If you're going to have a birthing pool, it's really worth doing a practice run, just so your partner knows what they're doing in terms of setting it up. Testing it out in advance is much less stressful than having to do it for the first time on the actual day, when there may be the distraction of you needing your partner's support, or labour progressing so fast that the pool isn't ready in time. It's useful to know beforehand how long it takes to inflate, how long it takes to fill, and whether your heating system is up to the job of delivering enough hot water for a nice, deep, warm pool of water when you need it.

- **What to do with your other children:**
  If this is not your first baby, you need to think about your plans for your other child(ren). First of all, do you want to have them there or do you feel that it might be distracting for you and/or upsetting for them? If the latter, in my experience it is, in fact, rare for children to get upset at a home birth. Women are usually very calm in their own environment, where they feel safe and focused. They don't tend to scream with the high-pitched sound of fear that's often heard on reality birth programmes;

they are much more likely to make low grunting sounds, synonymous with the effort involved, and children are quickly reassured if it is explained to them that this is the kind of noise Mummy has to make to help the baby come out. But it may be that, for you, it doesn't feel right. For example, you might feel that you cannot focus on the job in hand with your other child(ren) around; and, in the unlikely event that you have to transfer to an obstetric unit, you also have to consider who will stay behind with your children.

I was lucky enough to have Patti, my mother-in-law, on hand for all three of my home births. She lived in the basement of our house and was available 24/7 so the arrangement we had in place worked perfectly. When having Katie, my second baby, at home, I laboured in the daytime so Patti took Lucy, my eldest, out for a walk in the afternoon and came back to a new baby. My third and fourth births were both overnight labours – much more common – and we agreed that Patti would sit quietly by my bedroom door so that, if the children woke up and came in, they could either sit with her or, if they didn't want to stay or I didn't want them there, she would take them downstairs. In the event, neither of them woke up when Georgia was born, which was just before midnight. When they came in next morning, they were greeted with the sight of me peacefully breastfeeding their new little sister. The bonus that none of us had anticipated at the time was that for Patti, seeing the very straightforward and calm birth of her granddaughter was an unexpected healing experience for her after her own traumatic experience giving birth to Peter 34 years earlier.

Two years later, I also have the wonderful memory of my three little girls quietly pushing open my bedroom door literally moments after Arthur, my youngest son was born at around 7.10 on a beautiful summer's morning in 1991. They said hello to their brother amidst much excitement and then sat with Patti and watched in awe as I finished the work in hand and birthed the placenta!

Of course, whoever you ask to keep an eye on your children doesn't have to be someone who lives in your house. You might have family living nearby, or local friends or a neighbour who you can ask to be on standby. Make sure that all of the volunteers' contact numbers are in your partner's phone and that they understand they might get a call anytime, including the middle of the night. The circumstances may well be such that they'll need to come quickly, especially in the event of transfer.

• **What to expect/how labour might start:**
By this stage of your pregnancy, one hopes you will have got a sense of what you can expect from labour, either through classes, your own reading or the shared personal experiences of friends and family. There are, of course, as many different ways to labour as there are women, but there are some general principles that are useful to remember: one of the most important is pacing yourself through the latent or pre-labour phase, which can easily go on for a few days, especially with a first baby. Having realistic expectations and planning for how to cope with this early stage is key to staying calm and in tune with your body.

- **Contact numbers:**
Always make sure you have been given a number to contact to let someone know when you are in labour. Ideally, you will have a direct number for your midwife, but if not, check whether you have to ring the labour ward or the local triage or the community midwives' office. If you think your waters have broken, or you have any concerns, it can be very helpful to know you can ring your midwife and run them past her, usually for reassurance that all is well.

- **If no midwife is available on the day:**
You might also have to think about what you will do if you are told no midwife is available when you call. Unfortunately, this is not an isolated risk, especially in London and the bigger urban centres, because of the pressure on the service and a lack of midwives in general. The current situation is that, although your local health authority must provide a maternity service for the women in their area, they are not under a legal obligation to provide that service at your home. You also have a legal right, however, to choose where to have your baby, and midwives have a duty of care to attend a woman in labour, wherever they are. It is a good idea to have this conversation with your midwife well before you are due. If necessary, you might want to check what the policy is at the hospital where you are booked in. There are several organisations, such as the Association for Improvements in the Maternity Services (AIMS), Birthrights and the NCT who will offer you support and ideas about how to manage this situation if you find yourself faced with it.

- **Thinking about the choices you will need to make in labour:**
  The Birth Talk is an ideal opportunity – while you are relaxed and not having to deal with contractions – to discuss with your midwife your preferred choices about various aspects of labour. These will be specific to you but might include the following:

  - What your views are about vaginal examinations, the frequency they are offered, the reason for having them etc.
  - How you would like your baby's heartbeat to be monitored in labour and how often this will be offered.
  - Whether or not you would like to have a synthetic oxytocin injection (syntocinon) for the delivery of your placenta, with or without optimal cord clamping (allowing the blood flow between the placenta and new baby to continue, which improves neonatal iron stores).
  - If you would like your baby to have Vitamin K, which is recommended for all babies at birth, but, like everything else listed here, is your decision.

  All these things require informed consent from you before they can be carried out, and part of your planning for the day can include discussing these with your caregivers, who can record your decisions in your notes.

- **The immediate postnatal period:**
  Pregnancy is the perfect time to think about and plan for the first couple of weeks after your baby is born, which is usually the amount of time that partners can take off work. At the Birth Talk, I explain in some detail why it is

important to lay down some 'ground rules' for your family and friends *while you are pregnant* as it is much easier to get them to buy into the idea at this stage (rather than suddenly springing it on them once the baby is born) that you would rather they didn't visit for the first few days while you enjoy a 'babymoon'. Here are some suggestions:

* If this is your first baby, you could tell all your friends and family that you plan to have a quiet first few days with him or her and your partner (if you have one), just to recover from the labour and to enable breastfeeding to get off to a good start. There is nothing more calculated to start you on the slippery slope to exhaustion than to be waiting on a succession of visitors, especially if they are sitting there with your baby sleeping peacefully in their lap while you make endless cups of tea. You can explain very nicely that visitors will be very welcome on Day 4, or, if it is impossible to keep eager grandparents away, ask them if they can make the first visit short and sweet – ideally involving a meal that they have prepared and will clear up after! If you already have children, organising said friends and family to help look after your little ones is one very helpful contribution they can make to the post-baby planning phase.
* You can organise a big shop of non-perishable goods, prepare lots of delicious pre-cooked meals to keep in the freezer and generally be as organised as possible so that once the baby arrives you can do the first most important thing on my 'key principles' list: stay 'in bed' for the first week and spend the second week on the sofa! Before

you start worrying about getting a deep vein thrombosis (DVT) from lying around not moving, I hasten to add that you aren't necessarily in bed for the whole week, more that you stay in your pajamas and potter about in your bedroom, changing nappies in-between snoozing and feeding. Second key instruction: do not go downstairs to witness the bomb site your kitchen may or may not have become, depending on your partner's ability to keep the place tidy! There is time enough to put your home back in order – or you could ask an obliging grandparent to help – but don't go and look, especially if you know that you won't be able to resist starting to tidy up and clean.

- This time is precious and will very soon be over. It's the ideal opportunity to start to get to know this new little person in your life and, crucially, to tune in to their sleeping/waking cycles so that you can do the same (do not assume that you can go back to being awake all day, just like you normally do, and still cope after a busy night feeding).

Labour and Birth

What to Expect and How to Prepare

When describing the journey of labour and birth, it is very important to remember that although everyone talks about the 'stages' of labour and defines them as distinct and separate from each other, this is a relatively recent phenomenon and representative of the biomedical model rather than the more fluid and intuitive approach to the process that midwives used to rely on and which many still use to guide them in their observation and assessment of progress.

In a more holistic approach, labour and birth are seen as a continuum from late pregnancy through to the birth of the placenta. Although describing and timing the different stages can be used as a framework for discussion with your midwife, do keep in mind that this is merely a construct to try to define and understand the process rather than a hard-and-fast rule about how long any particular stage should last (or, indeed, that there is a cut-off point between them). There are national guidelines on the recommended length of each stage, depending on whether this is your first or a subsequent baby, but again they are only *guidelines*, so if, for example, you find things are progressing more slowly, don't feel pressurised into agreeing to a decision that really doesn't feel right for you.

Pre-labour

This refers to the period before the onset of labour. You may experience all or some of the 'symptoms' of pre-labour in a different way to other women, but they are usually present in some way, shape or form prior to the real thing!

In the weeks leading up to labour a series of processes start for both you and your baby that creates the conditions needed to stimulate and maintain labour. These processes are all inter-linked through complex hormonal activity and enable the uterus to move from its more passive role of housing your growing and developing baby to being in labour and actively flexing and contracting to birth him or her. Some of this hormonal activity includes the following:

- Progesterone levels, which inhibit uterine activity during pregnancy, begin to decrease, creating the necessary conditions for labour to begin.
- Maternal oestrogen increases, enabling the uterus to develop receptor sites – little pockets – to collect and hold oxytocin (*see* next bullet point).
- Oxytocin is key to a progressive and efficient labour. It is the hormone that produces and maintains effective con-tractions throughout the first, second and third stage of labour; then, after your baby is born, it helps your uterus

to shrink (involute), reinforces bonding and pushes milk through the breast to enable efficient and successful breast-feeding. Although oxytocin is produced naturally by the body, the artificial version (syntocinon) can also be given to augment labour or as an injection to help to deliver the placenta.

- There is a rise in the level of prostaglandins, which have a number of effects, including early changes to the cervix.
- Cortisol levels increase, which help to mature your baby's organs ready for labour and independent existence outside the womb.
- Endorphins are produced. These are the body's natural form of pain relief and produce a feeling of wellbeing. They are released in the weeks and days prior to labour to help the process along.
- Adrenalin is released. This stimulates the expulsive nature of contractions at the beginning of the second stage of labour but may also inhibit the production of oxytocin if levels get too high in early labour.

As the hormonal interplay gets going, you may begin to experience some cramping or 'tightening' of your uterus. This may be very mild or it can feel painful; it can be regular and may last for several hours at a time. It is very common to confuse these cramps as the start of labour proper and, since they often occur in the middle of the night, to make the mistake of getting up to breathe through them. Although trying to be 'active' is what is recommended to make labour more efficient, during pre-labour it is the quickest way to wear yourself out and get disheartened (i.e. after doing the same thing for one or two nights – or more – you can feel like you aren't getting anywhere and that your body isn't working properly).

In the overall context of birth, this phase is really important and, if you recognise it as pre-labour and relax into the sensations without trying to hurry them along, it can make the active phase more effective when it does eventually begin. So, how do you differentiate between the two? In my opinion the most important difference between pre-labour and active labour is a sense of progress. The sensations you experience in pre-labour usually all feel about the same strength and, even though they might be coming quite regularly, they just don't feel as if they are changing or progressing. This is in contrast to when labour is beginning to establish itself into the active phase and it gradually builds into a rhythm of regular contractions, which over a period of time get longer, stronger and more frequent.

If these tightenings come at night, try to ignore them as much as possible. Try to doze in-between them – often you will eventually drift off to sleep as they fade away. If they are impossible to manage in bed, you could run yourself a deep, warm bath to relax in ... this helps ease away the tension that often accompanies these unpleasant sensations, making them even more uncomfortable. If they come during the day, again try to ignore them as much as possible: live your life as normal, getting things ready for your baby, meeting up with friends etc. You can practise using your breath, or listen to hypnobirthing or relaxation tapes to manage the discomfort but try to remember that you are not in active labour and avoid the mistake of thinking that you are – it is then easier to pace yourself, be determined and remain emotionally strong. Remind yourself – and, most importantly, get others to remind you – that this is all normal: it is part of your body's preparation and you will go into labour eventually. There is a well-tested saying: 'If you have to ask yourself whether you are in labour, the answer is probably no!'

What is happening during the pre-labour phase?

All the hormones mentioned earlier are doing their bit to enable changes to take place that will eventually lead to labour starting. These include the changes below.

Cervical changes

The cervix is mostly comprised of connective tissue, covered with a thin layer of smooth muscle. In pregnancy, this connective tissue has a high level of collagen fibres, making the cervix feel firm (a bit like the end of your nose) and also helping to keep it tightly shut. During the period leading up to the onset of labour, there is a big reduction in the level of collagen and an increased vaginal watery discharge, which you will probably be aware of. For some women the quantity is considerable, making them think their membranes have broken and they are leaking amniotic fluid. If you are unsure, ask your midwife to check. The reason for this is that if your waters break and you don't go into labour within a certain time period, there is a recommendation to get labour started using drugs (augmentation) because of the small increased risk of infection. You will be asked to go into hospital for such a procedure – an unnecessary visit if it's only cervical changes.

During pregnancy, the cervix is normally in a posterior position, pointing backwards. This is so that, as the baby grows, their weight isn't directly over the cervix – which would put pressure on it and potentially increase the risk of premature delivery. Your cervix is about 3cm long, and has a tunnel or canal through the middle, with an inner and outer opening or 'os'. Sitting in the canal is thick mucus, known as the 'mucus plug', which helps to prevent infection during the months of pregnancy but may begin to come away as the cervix changes.

Part of the work being done by the cramping and tightenings in the uterus during the pre-labour phase is to begin to pull the cervix forward, while the prostaglandins are busy softening and thinning or 'effacing' it.

Positioning your baby

The other reason for regular tightenings during this pre-labour period is that your uterus might be trying to encourage your baby into a better position for the birth. For example, if your baby's head is not in your pelvis and you are experiencing lots of back ache, with most of your baby's movements being felt at the front of your abdomen, your baby may be in a posterior position (when their back is against your spine). In this position your baby is unable to easily move down or 'engage' in your pelvis because their head is not tucked in enough. If you suspect that might be the case, ask your midwife or GP to check at your next appointment.

It is useful to know this, because less-than-favourable positions can delay the onset of active labour or make the labour itself more challenging. This is particularly relevant if you are planning a home birth, so it is worth being pro-active and working with the tightenings to help your baby shift around.

Jean Sutton, a midwife from New Zealand, has written extensively about the value of 'optimal fetal positioning' (OFP) during the last weeks of pregnancy.[16] Her theory that the mother's position and movement during late pregnancy can influence the way her baby lies in the uterus is an interesting one, which I think has an instinctive element of common sense to it, although the evidence from one PhD research study has not confirmed her theory.[17]

Whatever the arguments for or against, adopting certain positions in late pregnancy is unlikely to do you any harm, as long as you keep a reasonable perspective on it all. During this period, try to keep upright and reasonably mobile. If possible, avoid spending ages sitting in a car or in low chairs with your knees higher than your hips, which may encourage the baby's back to rotate into a less favourable position ... turning a dining chair around and sitting on it back to front with your legs open and tummy forward, for example, also helps to keep the weight of the baby over the cervix as it becomes more central. This then increases the release of prostaglandins – which in turn helps the softening process – a feedback mechanism that is a great example of just how clever your body is!

Good positions for late pregnancy

The onset of labour

There are no rules that govern whether or not you have a long, short or non-existent pre-labour phase: it varies from woman to woman and from one pregnancy to another. The best thing to do is to go with the flow and stay as calm and relaxed as possible whatever the challenges of this period. It can feel like a very long time, especially if you are constantly being asked by well-meaning friends and relatives if you have had the baby yet … so practising patience and trying to stay in the moment are useful skills to develop, while you await the onset of labour itself.

However, if this pre-labouring activity is happening of its own accord but taking you past your due date, you may also want to think about some additional activities to encourage things to move on. You will find a few suggestions under the postdates section (*see* page 135).

First stage labour: cervical dilation and the descent of your baby

Early labour/latent phase

This is the early phase of the first stage of labour and describes the period of time it takes for the cervix to become thinned out or 'fully effaced' and to reach about 4cm dilation. You will usually experience mild to moderate contractions of the uterus, which will vary in how painful they feel and will tend to be irregular in timing and length. Early labour feels different to pre-labour in that, although the contractions are not yet regular, they tend not to stop and start; also, although they are usually manageable, they can feel more painful than pre-labour tightenings, sometimes considerably so.

Once contractions have been going on for a few hours, women who are having a planned hospital birth have to start trying to work out when to go to the labour ward, which can be the start of a slippery slope. Looked at logically, it doesn't seem to make sense to recommend that women in the throes of labour should get into a car, drive to an unfamiliar environment and enter a busy labour ward with its noise, activity, commotion and strangers, just at the point when they should be settling into the active part of their labour, feeling safe and surrounded by familiar faces.

It's extremely rare in today's maternity services, because of the way they are currently organised, for a woman to have a midwife she has already met care for her on the labour ward. This can impact in a number of different ways: established labour can be very difficult to define or categorise, especially if you are seeing lots of different midwives who may all have their own interpretation. You may not get a consistent view as to exactly where you are on the labour journey, even with a vaginal examination to assess progress. Most midwifery knowledge is subjective and there are very few definitively right or wrong answers. That is why it can be very helpful to have just one or two midwives look after you throughout your pregnancy with whom you can build a relationship of trust. Having the same midwife assessing your progress during your labour reduces the chance of different interpretations, even if it doesn't entirely rule out the occasional 'misdiagnosis' of established labour.

The other reason why consistency of care matters is that when labouring women find themselves in situations where they become distressed or fearful, they produce hormones that can be counterproductive to giving birth. The neocortex (our 'thinking brain') will also become highly active instead of being 'switched off' during labour because it is stimulated when we have to answer complicated questions, are exposed to bright lights, are feeling vulnerable or are aware of being watched and feel as if we need to stay on guard. If a woman is anxious, frightened, scared, angry or embarrassed, her levels of catecholamines and cortisol, which are adrenaline-based hormones (the 'stress hormones'), will be too high. This can have the effect of switching off the oxytocin and endorphins that are naturally produced through labour, thereby possibly reducing the chances of maintaining straightforward progress and even stopping labour.

Labours that slow down are very common in labour wards. In addition to what is termed 'failure to progress', fear and tension increase, both of which cause labour to be more painful than it needs to be. This cycle of events can be why, when a woman moves from her quiet, personal space at home to a busy, bustling labour ward, she is more likely to need her labour to be 'augmented' because it has slowed down or to need pain relief because of the effect on her ability to manage the intensity of her contractions.

Trisha Anderson's article 'Out of the laboratory: back to the darkened room' uses a wonderful analogy of how cats birth.[18] Cats will only labour and birth in a calm space in the furthest corner of the darkest room; if you disturb them, the labour will stop and they will become distressed, as will the kittens. In Anderson's dystopian vision, scientists observe cats giving birth in a lab over many years, and unsurprisingly, they start to have increasingly more dysfunctional, erratic labours that stop and start, with the effect that their kittens are traumatised at birth. So the scientists begin to give pain relief to the cats to relieve their symptoms and thereby try to reduce the effects of having brought them into the lab in the first place.

Unfortunately, we have inadvertently created the same environment for labouring women. We have forgotten that women actually birth better when left alone in a supported, calm, quiet and safe space – one that they feel is their own. Healthy women with well-grown, healthy babies are perfectly adapted to giving birth in the peace and quiet of their own space. However, we began to encourage them to leave it because everyone made the erroneous assumption that it would be safer to be near doctors, in a place where they could be helped if things went wrong. It didn't seem to occur to anyone that this strategy might actually be creating the very problems we were trying to avoid. The difficulty now is that this has become normalised – there have already been a few generations of midwives working in this environment and women giving birth in this way.

One of the many advantages to planning a home birth is that once you think labour has started you can contact your midwife and she will come out to assess you at home, rather than you needing to go anywhere – usually the labour ward – to have your progress confirmed, or not! Going to a labour ward for this purpose is often a time-consuming, exhausting process that can result in several back-and-forth trips if you are deemed to be less than 3–4cm dilated and therefore not in 'established' labour. This scenario is much more common with first babies, but even if you have had a baby before, it can be very frustrating not to know if you are dilated enough to be admitted into the birth centre or labour ward. To be honest, as we've just discussed, it's not in your best interests to be admitted too early, as managing early labour, especially if you have prepared well, is better done within the comfort and privacy of your own home, whether or not you choose to birth your baby there.

Depending on where you live and what the different options are for your maternity care, some midwifery teams may include the option of a home assessment, even if you plan to transfer once in established labour, so it is worth asking if that is available when making your choices. It may not seem very relevant when you are only a few weeks pregnant, but it can make the difference between a calmer, more relaxed start to your labour or a more fraught and stressed one.

How contractions work

In the last weeks of pregnancy and continuing into early labour, the cells that make up the uterus develop an increasing number of protein units between them, known as 'gap junctions'. These can be found in any tissue that needs to act in a coordinated way, such as cardiac muscle. The little channels or junctions connect two cells together and increase the communication between them – in this way, a contraction in one cell is communicated and passed on to the next so that eventually every contraction becomes synchronised and the uterus contracts in a harmonised, coordinated way.

However, the uterus also needs coordination between its upper and lower half, known as 'polarity'. In labour, the upper half contracts and retracts – which is a unique property of uterine muscle. When the contraction ends, the muscle fibres don't completely relax back to their original state; and so over the course of the labour, they gradually shorten and thicken, pulling up the lower half of the uterus, which is simultaneously contracting, relaxing and gradually dilating. The upper and lower segments have to work in harmony with each other, with the peak of the contraction being reached at the same time across the whole uterus, in order for labour to progress.

The cervix, which, as it thins out eventually becomes part of the lower segment of the uterus, is situated within many layers of muscle fibres and tissue. The more tense and anxious we are in labour, the more painful the contraction is likely to feel as the tension is held in the pelvic area and may inhibit the ability of the lower segment to relax and dilate in-between contractions.

Established labour/active phase

This is usually recognised as the onset of regular, long, strong and frequent contractions and will generally be diagnosed by your midwife following a vaginal examination to assess dilatation and effacement of your cervix. By the time you are in established labour, particularly if this is your first baby, you may have been having contractions (*see* page 169) for many hours or even days. This is why it is so important to pace yourself and plan, with your birth partner(s) and midwife, how and by whom you will be supported, including regular food and drink, rest/sleep, change of scene/activity, baths and/or showers, regular trips to the loo. ABOVE ALL ELSE, staying in the moment, managing each contraction as it comes, working with it and not getting too far ahead in your mind are crucial to successfully pacing yourself.

Don't allow the idea to take hold that you can't do any more, especially after a particularly strong contraction. Labour is as much, if not more, about your psychological and emotional resilience as it is about the physical stamina everyone focuses on. Although the latter is important, the reality is that nearly all women can manage that side of it … lots of second, third and fourth winds help, and you need to keep reminding yourself that women are made to have babies, we are actually very good at it – we've just forgotten that we are and we've lost the key ingredient ... continuous support from known and trusted birth partners. You will need to plan during your pregnancy who will be there for you when you need some external input. This needs to be positive energy, because if anyone starts doubting your ability, it can be the start of a slippery slope where your own sense of 'I know I can do this' begins to question itself.

It is important to note here that there is a difference between the power of a normal labour and a labour that is dysfunctional or not progressing normally. Sometimes you might feel instinctively that something isn't quite right and, if that is the case it is always important to check that out with your midwife to see if it is confirmed by any of her observations and monitoring.

Transition

This describes a phase of labour that lots of women have heard about as being the time when you might want to call the whole thing off or you start swearing like a trooper at your husband! It's usually towards the end of the first stage of labour, when you are nearing full dilation and your body is beginning to ready itself for pushing your baby out into the world. The best explanation I've heard for why transition happens and why it can be difficult to manage is that, after having got into a nice rhythm with first stage contractions, managing them well, breathing through and being very focused and then resting or getting your breath back in-between, your body starts to send out two rather conflicting messages: one tells you that the energy flow is still overwhelmingly upwards, pulling open the cervix and thinning out the lower segment of the uterus to create the space for the baby to move down into the vagina. But then, as the baby begins to move down on to the pelvic floor, using gravity and being squeezed by the contractions, the energy flow starts to change and is redirected downwards, prior to the expulsive pushing of the second stage. Your rhythm can get lost in these conflicting messages, which can upset the calm focus of earlier contractions, and suddenly you start questioning your ability to cope with the more unpredictable nature of the sensations and messages circulating in your body.

Should this happen to you – and transition is not a universal experience – the most important thing to remember is that it means you are progressing well and that the end, if not imminent, is at least now in sight.

The benefits of being at home, as well as the feeling of safety and comfort that is there automatically, can really come into their own during what can be a very challenging time in your labour. You are supported by your environment, not restricted by it as you would be in hospital or a birth centre where you can't suddenly decide to change rooms or you are attached to a monitor, or have an intravenous (IV) solution or a catheter inserted, for example. If you reach a point when you feel as if you can't keep going, or an epidural (a local anaesthetic injected into the epidural space of the spinal column) and even a caesarean section suddenly seem like a really good idea, changing the energy in the room, heading out into the garden, for example, or going to sit on your own loo can really help divert your thoughts. You can then refocus as the labour moves on and you either begin to spontaneously push or have a 'rest-and-be-thankful' phase (when the contractions can space out and give you a bit of a breathing space before the second stage kicks in).

Second stage: birthing your baby

Personally, I love the second stage! During my labours, it felt as if I was now actively working with my contractions, rather than just having to cope with them, which is how dilation or the first stage of labour can sometimes feel. However, with a first baby, the time needed to push him or her down the birth canal can sometimes feel like an eternity. This is when having that quiet, tireless support and encouragement of your birth partners and midwives can really make a difference. Sometimes it can take just a few pushes, especially for a second or subsequent baby, but often that short distance your baby has to travel can feel like an impossibly long way.

You may be feeling tired and a little disheartened by the hours of work you have already put into birthing your little one, but at some point you will begin to spontaneously start pushing as the process of labour moves into its expulsive phase. This is often the time when you can get a second (or it might be your third or fourth) wind, a renewed sense of purpose and a growing excitement – or perhaps slight trepidation – that your baby is on the way. If you are in water, moving around into different positions can be managed very easily. But if you are on solid ground, it can be really helpful to change positions whenever it feels as if progress has slowed or you are tiring.

You and your baby are a team, working together to bring him or her into the world. It can be surprising how effective it can be to go from kneeling to putting one foot up, or turning around into a deep squat to bring your baby around the bend of the pubic symphysis. Some women will move instinctively, but others can get a little 'stuck' and that is when your midwife might quietly suggest a change of position to keep the momentum up and help move your baby down.

If it feels right, a favourite tip to try is to head out to the loo (which is where the tea trays have come in useful on more than one occasion). If you have been standing or kneeling and your legs are tiring, sitting on the loo with them nice and wide apart can be restful – it's also where women can sometimes relax into more effective pushing as it feels so familiar to do that there.

The one place you probably won't choose if at home, or at least not to lie down on, is the bed. It is very rare that women head there when the birth is imminent, although it might still occasionally be suggested by your midwife, especially if she is more used to working in a hospital setting than in a woman's home environment. As we have all seen on our TV screens, through programmes like *One Born Every Minute*, it is still almost automatic in an obstetric labour ward for women to be directed towards the bed, often to end up on their back, or equally unhelpfully, sitting on their coccyx. I have also heard, from anecdotal conversations with student midwives, that lithotomy (your legs being put up in stirrups as you lie flat on your back) as a position for women supposedly having a normal labour is becoming more common again. Lying on your side, though, in what is known as the 'left lateral position', can give you a rest if you have been on your knees for a while and can be very effective at moving your baby through the birth canal.

By and large, at some point in the second stage of labour you will probably find yourself in the positions that have proved themselves over the millennia as the best at harnessing the power of gravity: squatting, kneeling or sitting. You can pull back from strong banisters or bed boards and use every-day household objects or special aids such as birth balls and stools for support … it's your call and you might find that you make use of most of them at some point during this phase.

Second stage is also where the last few weeks of practice with an Epi-No® comes into its own. Many women tighten their muscles almost by reflex as the baby's head moves down because they feel as if they are either going to do a poo or break wind and we are very conditioned not to do either in 'public' or away from the toilet. Using the Epi-No in late pregnancy prepares that whole area and gets you used to the sensations of opening and stretching', so that when it is happening for real you stay nice and soft and relaxed and don't fight them or instinctively clench your muscles. Should you happen to pass a small bowel movement, your midwife will be completely unfazed and indeed will often be very pleased as it is usually a sure sign that the baby is not far away now.

The crowning of the baby's head, that point of no return just before the head is born, will be something of a test for many women, causing as it often does the 'ring of fire' or burning sensation as the skin and tissue stretch and give, one hopes without tearing. Trusting the process and using your breath to pant the baby over the perineum, perhaps in conjunction with a lovely hot compress (another – literally – hot tip that is so much easier to organise at home). A recently boiled kettle can keep the hot water topped up in a bowl and most women love the sensation of the hot flannel against their perineum. And, then, before you know it, your baby is born and in your arms, either passed through your legs by your midwife if you are kneeling, or scooped up by you if in the pool.

Holding this space, this very special moment when you and your partner are greeting your baby for the first time, is such a privilege for us as midwives, sitting back and quietly observing or perhaps taking photos or doing whatever might have been discussed and agreed previously. I am always in awe at the strength and extraordinary power of women in this moment, a feeling that has only grown stronger over all the years I've been working as a midwife. I think it's partly due to the deep pleasure of seeing women in their own environment, responding to the moment in whatever way feels right – because they are in their own home, what they do in it is entirely up to them.

Facilitating immediate skin to skin, in other words you and your baby having a cuddle, is now pretty much routine wherever you have your baby, unless for some reason he or she needs to be taken away from you briefly to be checked over. Most mothers will instinctively pick up or receive their babies into their arms and will then bring them to their breast, sometimes after needing a few moments of letting the reality that their baby is actually here sink in.

Cardinal movements of labour

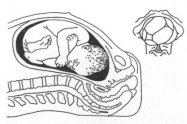 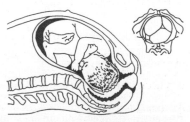

Head floating, before engagement   Engagement; descent, flexion

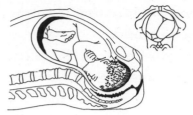

Further descent, internal rotation

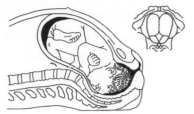
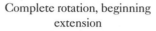

Complete rotation, beginning
extension

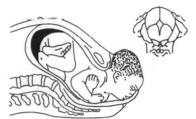

Complete extension

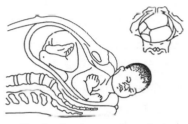

Restitution (external rotation)

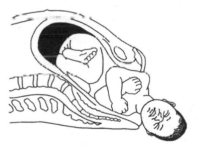

Delivery of anterior shoulder

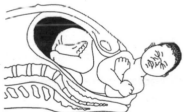

Delivery of posterior shoulder

Third stage: birthing your placenta

Another reason for all the lovely warm feelings usually felt by
everyone present is that we're probably all a little high on
oxytocin. It makes me think of Titania in Shakespeare's
Midsummer Night's Dream and the magical juice concocted
from the flower 'love-in-idleness', which, when applied to the

eyelids of a sleeping person, causes that person, upon waking, to fall in love with the first living thing they see.

The French obstetrician Michel Odent coined the phrase 'oxytocin is the hormone of love', mainly because it is the hormone linked to orgasm as well as birth. Soon after your baby is born, your body, in an unmedicated labour, will produce a large surge of oxytocin. The physiological impact of this is to produce a nice big contraction, which will usually ensure that the placenta is sheared off the uterine wall, ready to slip through the cervix and eventually be pushed out through the birth canal. The by-product of this big surge of the 'love hormone' is that, as you are meeting your baby, often oblivious to what is going on internally, the oxytocin will reinforce the bonding process: as you gaze at the new love in your life, your feelings towards this little person are intensified and strengthened. It's just another clever way that Nature has of maximising the chances of bonding kicking in with the birth of your baby. It isn't failsafe, of course, and, depending on what sort of pregnancy you've had and what else is going on in your life, it may be that the bonding doesn't happen immediately.

The key thing to keep in the back of your mind during these first magical moments after your baby is born is that just because the baby is here it doesn't mean that labour is over. Until the placenta is out and the third stage complete, it is important to keep the same atmosphere as for the birth (i.e. usually quiet and private with dim lighting) and – very important – a warm room temperature to help maintain the hormonal activity needed to conclude the process.

This is all much easier to do in your own space of course, especially if you've had an opportunity to talk about this time during the pregnancy Birth Talk. However, there is sometimes a temptation to start phoning around or inviting lots of family into the room to share the wonderful news. While this is a lovely thing to do, ideally it's best done after the placenta is out and your midwife is happy that the blood loss is not too much and that there are no immediate clinical issues that might need to be dealt with.

Many women choosing to birth at home, especially if they are planning not to use any, or only minimal, pain relief, will also be interested in choosing a *physiological third stage* (i.e. one without the use of any oxytocic drugs, allowing the cord to pulsate until it naturally finishes and then pushing out the placenta through their own effort and without the midwife doing anything physical other than observing and monitoring blood loss). The midwife may give lots of guidance, including suggestions of different positions and general support, but it is crucial that she does not pull on the cord or interfere with the placenta in any way. (It is often the mixing up of the two methods used to birth or deliver the placenta that can cause problems rather than a physiological approach being inherently more risky.)

The alternative to this is an *active or managed third stage*, when your midwife will give you an injection and then await the signs of separation, which are usually a small gush or trickle of blood and a lengthening of the cord, after which she will deliver the placenta by gently but firmly pulling on the cord, while simultaneously protecting or 'guarding' your uterus.

Although a physiological third stage is usually a slightly longer process then an actively managed one, being focused on any returning contractions and being proactive about working with them and actively pushing when the sensations come, will help ensure it doesn't end up taking hours rather than the 20–40 minutes the third stage should last. Encouraging your baby to explore your breast and nipple, while he or she is cradled in your arms or lying on your chest, can also help, as the continued production of oxytocin that results from the stimulation of your breasts also reminds your uterus it still has a job to do in expelling the placenta.

Another option is to head off to the loo again, this time with a bowl placed inside to catch the placenta on its way out. Sometimes just the act of getting upright and moving will encourage the placenta to begin its journey; and once you are on the loo, the same instinct to relax and push kicks in, and out will slide your placenta. You can also hold your breath and then blow into a bottle or against your closed fist to create the pressure that helps to push the placenta down through the folds of your vaginal walls. (On a trip to Zimbabwe with my family back in 1999, I spent a wonderful afternoon in the warm, sunny backyard of a local health clinic, talking with a group of midwives. As we compared the differences in midwifery practice between our two cultures, we also realised how many similarities there were, especially in home birth scenarios, one of which was the use of a bottle to encourage the placenta out!)

In most cases of physiological birth, the placenta separates within the first few minutes after the cord has stopped pulsating, and the chances are that it is just sitting there waiting for you to push it out. So I always think it's worth being upright and letting the combination of gravity and a bit of maternal effort get the job done sooner rather than later.

Although many people are a little squeamish about it, to me the placenta is a rather beautiful object, as well as being a complex and extraordinary life-support organ. One of the things I love to do when I am getting ready to examine it after a birth is to explain how it worked, how the baby was inside the membranes and where the exit hole is, and to show the new parents how the placenta looks like the tree of life, with the umbilical cord as the trunk and all the blood vessels that run through it like the branches. It is also, of course, yours to keep and, while we are happy to take it away if that is your choice, you do also have the option of popping it into the freezer for burying out in the garden another day ... perhaps with a specially chosen tree or bush planted with it. There are also other options – placental encapsulation (a process in which your placenta is dehydrated and ground into a coarse powder) and placenta smoothies to name but two – the choice is yours!

Perineal care and suturing at home

Labour is done, your baby may or may not have fed yet, and it might be before or after your lovely welcome bath, but at some point your midwife will ask if she can examine your perineum and vagina to see whether or not you have suffered a tear. In the unlikely event that you have had an episiotomy at home, she will know that you will need stitches to repair it, but either way, a careful and thorough examination is essential to confirm the presence of any laceration, how extensive it is and whether or not stitches – or 'sutures' as they are known – are advised.

The evidence is still somewhat inconclusive about whether or not to suture. The current advice is that while first-degree tears, which involve only the skin, are okay to leave, midwives should be cautious about leaving second-degree tears, which involve the muscle, unsutured.[19] It is, however, always your decision, and a full and thorough discussion should take place at the time to enable you to make as fully informed a choice as possible and one that feels right for you and your circumstances. (For more information, visit www.rcm.org.uk/sites/default/files/Suturing the Perineum.pdf.)

Ideally, this discussion has been initiated during the pregnancy and the topic revisited by your midwife during the Birth Talk, so that if she is going to be the midwife at your birth, she will know what your preferences are. Otherwise, try to ensure that you have the conversation at some point during your pregnancy and then consider including your preferences in a written birth plan so that the midwife at your birth can refer to it.

As in all things birth-related, there are lots of different considerations to take into account before an individual decision is made. General health and wellbeing are a major consideration because healthy tissue will heal better, and certain lifestyle choices, such as smoking, impact heavily on tissue health and repair.

You need to be honest with yourself and your midwife about whether or not you will be able to, or perhaps more to the point, you will choose to rest well after birth. Will you follow the 'one week in bed, one week on the sofa' rule (mentioned on page 58 as a crucial element of the postnatal period, which ideally should be planned for well in advance) or will you be running up and down stairs from Day 2? If you think you are more likely to be in the latter category, you should seriously consider having stitches in order to maximise the chances of keeping the two opposing sides of the tear together while they mend.

If, however, you are going to be conscientious about resting properly, eating really well (food that has been prepared by your carers), doing your pelvic floor exercises (which encourage healthy blood flow and aid healing) and not rushing around, not sitting cross-legged and trying to avoid picking up your sturdy two-year-old the whole time, chances are a straightforward second-degree tear that sits together well, isn't bleeding and is not too extensive, will probably heal well – albeit perhaps more slowly than a sutured tear, but possibly with less discomfort and swelling.

If the decision is made to suture, an experienced home birth midwife will be very adept at utilising your furniture, creating a temporary clinical space with you on the edge of the bed and your feet up on two stools, for example. Then, she will either use a head torch, or a second midwife will hold one; or, if you have one, an Anglepoise lamp can be positioned to ensure a clear, well-lit view of the perineum.

If your midwife has any doubts about the wisdom of trying to suture a more complex or deeper tear at home, she will discuss with you the need for transfer into your local obstetric unit to have a review or, at the very least, to enable a more thorough examination, perhaps with more effective pain relief. You should always be offered local anaesthesia by injection before suturing starts; you can also go back to using gas and air (Entonox®) during the procedure, but even with that it is not the most comfortable process, especially if it is coming at the end of a long and tiring labour when you just want to climb into bed.

There are many helpful strategies you will be able to put in place to help avoid tearing or the need for an episiotomy. Using the Epi-No®, perineal massage, doing regular pelvic floor exercises, having a good diet and taking regular exercise during pregnancy, plus a physiological approach to the second stage of labour, can work wonders. In the second stage it is especially important to work with your body's messages – in tune with the pushing sensations and with none of the 'directed pushing' or cheerleading from your caregivers that evidence shows has a potentially negative effect on your baby's health (it doesn't allow for gentle, gradual stretching, with the baby rocking back and forth, which is Nature's way of protecting your birth canal and perineum).[20]

When these strategies are combined with some helpful guidance from your midwife as you breathe your baby gently out over the perineum, either in water, which provides a protective element or with a hot compress in place, the chances are greatly increased that you will have either an intact perineum or only a minor tear.

Pain Relief at Home

By choosing a home birth, you are also making a choice about restricting or limiting the choices of pain relief open to you, which is one of the many reasons you might be questioned on your sanity for making this choice. An epidural is not an option at home so if you want one, you will need to transfer to an obstetric unit. It is really important to emphasise that if you do decide to transfer for that reason, you have not 'failed' in any way. Such unnecessary judgement is deeply unhelpful because sometimes labours are best managed with this form of pain relief, especially if the baby is not in a great position, or your contractions are not consistently strong enough to open the cervix and you have been labouring for many hours without progress.

These things happen and sometimes labour takes an unexpected turn and you might need to rethink your 'Plan A' for all sorts of reasons. I think that part of your decision-making about where to have your baby really needs to include this element – being very open and honest with yourself and others, especially if this is your first baby, about not necessarily knowing how you will cope with and respond to the contractions you are given.

In my experience, women who have transferred to an obstetric unit for additional pain relief rarely regret the time they have spent labouring at home. They usually feel very positive about their labour and birth experience because it's still them in the driving seat, making the decision about when to transfer and having a very clear sense of the reasons why. We will have talked about the possibility during the pregnancy and about keeping an open mind on what you might decide to do once you are in the reality of the labour. It is really not something to waste a moment beating yourself up about!

Having said that, and returning to the theme running throughout this book, before we explore what sort of pain relief is available at home, it is useful to remind ourselves that women, in common with most other female mammals, will generally experience straightforward and uncomplicated labours when they feel safe and secure, are supported by people they trust and can be relaxed in their own environment.

Labour can risk becoming dysfunctional when you are planning to have your baby in an obstetric unit birth and have to leave your warm and safe environment to drive there. This may be at night but can sometimes be through busy streets and rush-hour traffic; your nearest obstetric unit may be handling up to 5,000 births a year and so will invariably be a place of bustle, noise, lights and lots of people you have never met before ... the very things that we now know are more likely to put you off your stride and slow labour down.

Two typical scenarios

Scenario 1

You are labouring well at home, contracting every three minutes, getting into 'the zone' and beginning to feel like things are really happening ... your partner may have tried ringing the hospital a few times and been put off, but eventually you are invited to come in and arrive there after an uncomfortable and stressful journey (no one wants to be having strong contractions in a moving car).

Upon arriving at the hospital you might be greeted by a midwife who is having a long and stressful day of her own and is perhaps not as kind or as patient as she could be. As your anxiety begins to build, adrenaline and cortisol begin to pump through your system, which is one of the most effective ways to switch off oxytocin, sometimes called the 'shy' hormone because of its tendency to disappear in the presence of catecholamines such as adrenaline, which are released into your bloodstream at times of physical or emotional stress. You wait ages to be seen, by which time you realise that your contractions have dwindled away – they have lost their intensity and the nice rhythm you were in at home. You are eventually examined and are only 2–3cm dilated, with irregular or sporadic contractions and so are not deemed to be in established labour.

You are sent home, where you find it much more difficult to get back into the flow, and feel anxious and tense. As a result, when the contractions do come, they are sharp and much more uncomfortable and you don't seem able to get on top of them.

Eventually, you head back to the hospital, possibly because you are not coping with the pain in the same way as before and are really struggling to keep going. If you still haven't progressed – which, in spite of what feels like intense pain, is entirely possible because you might by now be very tense and the contractions may be uncoordinated – you might end up being admitted to the antenatal ward to be given pethidine (an opiate-based pain relief given by injection) because you can't face the journey home again and insist on staying. All of this is exhausting and draining … not the best start to your labour journey!

Scenario 2

Contrast that scenario with how things usually unfold with a planned home birth. It is a very different story because you have removed one of the main reasons why so many women may get anxious and tense in labour – trying to decide when is the right time to go into hospital and what will happen when they get there. It is this growing tension that can make the contractions so much more unbearable and difficult to cope with. Staying in your known, safe and private space helps you maintain a relaxed state of mind and, therefore, a relaxed physical state, which will help to prevent your muscles and tissues from tensing up and feeling increasingly tight and uncomfortable – even when there is no contraction there. With no other distractions, you can get into your rhythm, and your birth partner can focus on you, reminding you when necessary, with a gentle word or touch, to let go of your breath at the end of a contraction. As you do so, your shoulders relax, your jaw unclenches and your hands let go of whatever they were gripping!

By the time the next contraction starts to build, you are relaxed, focused and ready to breathe your way through it again … and so you go on through your labour, one contraction at a time.

Top techniques for relieving pain

Using your breath

There are a variety of techniques and options available to you during your pregnancy that are all related to the ability, through practice, to switch off your active 'thinking' mind and harness the power of the breath. In my experience, breathing mindfully and in the moment is one of the simplest and most useful 'interventions' at our disposal during labour and birth.

All of us breathe involuntarily and usually without conscious thought – that's how we stay alive – but holding our breath can also be an unconscious response to painful stimuli, and that is not helpful in labour. If you bang your shin or stub your toe, you will often grit your teeth and hold your breath, managing the pain that way. But, when you are in the middle of a contraction, holding your breath will usually make the pain worse by increasing and holding the tension in that area.

It never ceases to amaze me just what an effective form of pain relief breathing out slowly and mindfully, with your conscious focus on that outward breath, can be. It can really help you to stay in control and on top of the pain, working with it instead of trying to get away from it. I have a vivid memory from my own labours of how, whenever I started to struggle with the intensity of a particular contraction, the sound of my birth partner, Christine, breathing out next to me and encouraging me to tune into her rhythm helped me to reconnect with my own breath and stop the mounting panic from overwhelming me.

There are lots of different examples of how you can work with your breath. It is worth spending some time researching some of them to find one that works for you and then practise it regularly throughout your pregnancy.

Hypnosis, hypnobirthing and natal hypnotherapy

Hypnobirthing and natal hypnotherapy are both terms you may come across if you are researching the use of hypnosis in pregnancy and labour. They are similar in that they both use professional hypnosis techniques to teach how relaxation, hypnosis and reducing fear can help manage the pain in labour. However, there are some differences: hypnobirthing is from the United States and is more prescriptive, with set visualisations and pre-recorded CDs, whereas natal hypnotherapy is a more individualised course, with the focus on your unique experience and situation and adapting words and scripts for each woman.

Both require practice throughout the pregnancy, although the hypnobirthing version relies on and expects the partner to be involved, whereas natal hypnotherapy can be done by the woman on her own. Often these things come down to individual preferences and finding out what works for you.

During hypnobirthing classes, you learn about the effect of accumulating fear and anxiety on the hormonally driven fight, flight or freeze responses. Once you are aware of this, you can override the response and choose to stay calm, so reducing the pain that is associated with fear and tension. It takes practice to learn the calming techniques required to increase the release of endorphins and avoid the constricting effect of negative hormones, but over time the life skills you learn can be used in many different situations.

Self-hypnosis is increasingly seen as a very effective tool for managing the pain of labour, and there is a choice of more and more classes and teachers. If I'm honest though, I do worry sometimes that some of the hypnobirthing videos I've seen, which show women breathing their baby out silently and without any signs of discomfort, may inadvertently set women up to fail.

My own experience over the years of how women cope with labour is that it can often require some serious noises to aid effort: grunting, bellowing, whatever it takes! The important thing here is that there is no one 'correct' way. Noisy births and quiet births are both entirely valid, and the likelihood is that by practising these techniques during pregnancy you are going to feel more able to be spontaneous with what works for you in labour.

Talking of being noisy in labour, if you are worried about what the neighbours might think, have a word with them before your due date and let them know that if they hear anything, not to worry as it will just be you in labour! Interestingly, neighbours often don't hear much, perhaps because the sounds that women naturally make in labour tend to be much lower in pitch than what you might be used to hearing on TV progammes involving labour wards. The sounds that women make in those environments are often quite high-pitched, fear-based screams, whereas the grunting noises I'm describing are more to do with effort.

Mindfulness and meditation

Mindfulness and meditation techniques have become very popular in recent years, and pregnancy is a perfect opportunity to start practising them. This is because we tend to feel vulnerable during this time and are open to finding positive ways of responding to discomfort and negative thoughts and emotions.

Mindfulness is a mental state achieved by focusing one's awareness on the present moment, while calmly acknowledging and accepting the transient flow of feelings, thoughts, and bodily sensations. It takes a great deal of practice, but by working on being fully present – not forcing things or hiding from them, but actually being with them – we can create space to respond in new ways to challenging situations.

Pregnancy yoga

Taking up or continuing to do yoga is one of the best preparations you can do in pregnancy, both for your own wellbeing and for your baby. There are lots of different classes around, so find one that suits you, making sure that you always listen to your body and don't overdo any of the exercises or stretching.

Practising yoga regularly throughout pregnancy develops your stamina and strength, especially in your back and hips. It helps you with your balance and can relieve tension in your back, shoulders and anywhere else it collects.

During labour, the practice of using and working with your breath, which is the foundation of yoga, can come into its own, helping to manage the pain of each contraction while maintaining your calm and reducing the tension and fear associated with pain.

Massage

Massage as a form of pain relief works not only on a physical level by reducing muscular tension, but also helps to reduce the stress associated with pain by releasing serotonin and endorphins. In the absence of a skilled massage therapist, this is something your partner can learn to do during your pregnancy and labour. Using firm rhythmic strokes can really help alleviate lower back pain, for example, and the effect of 'skin to skin' can also help oxytocin levels. Although there isn't a great deal of evidence in this area, what there is suggests a positive effect on pain management in labour.[21]

Sophrology and visualisation

Relatively new to this country, sophrology describes a set of dynamic exercises designed to help you be more relaxed, mindful and serene. It doesn't just apply to pregnancy and birth although it lends itself particularly well to this key life event. A sophrology practitioner will teach you different movements, visualisations and postures to explore your own particular issues and to practise in your own time.

Riding the wave

The range of different coping behaviours is wide and you may be able to dip in and out of several or be very focused on one particular technique. But whatever you choose, practising it throughout your pregnancy is really important.

This is because our natural response to pain tends to be that we tense up and grit our teeth, so we have to try to be counter-intuitive in our response during labour, welcoming each contraction and preparing to ride with it, almost like bodysurfing a wave, breathing smoothly and in tune with it, not fighting it or holding our breath.

If you've been practising all your chosen methods of relaxation during pregnancy – mindfulness, yoga, meditation, breathing and hypnobirthing, for example, it enables you to develop a different response when the pain starts to kick in. To continue with the example of the beginning of a contraction, as it begins to build, our mind recognises it as something familiar and can then override the instinctive response, which is to pull away from the pain, to tense up and hold our breath. If instead we can stay calm and relaxed, we will usually manage the contractions better and the likely effect of that is that our need for pain relief is greatly reduced.

Of course, sometimes labour can become more difficult to deal with because of other factors such as the position of the baby (the classic example is where he or she is back to back or posterior). But in the case of normal labour, with a reasonably well-positioned baby, understanding and being able to manage the contractions in this way will give you a great feedback mechanism: as you put your strategies into effect and realise the benefit you are getting from them, it creates a positive loop that can override the negative one telling you that the pain is too much, and can help make you more determined to stay the course.

If you have worked your way through all the pros and cons about where to have your baby and you've made the decision to have a home birth, then the likelihood is that you've thought about pain relief and how you might be able to manage the labour without medication. When labour starts, therefore, you are less likely to get into the spiral of tension that leads to increased pain. By maximising your chances of staying relaxed and feeling serene and secure – not anxious or scared – you have an added advantage right from the word 'go'.

Natural pain relief

Endorphins

We're back to hormones and the amazing effect of endorphins (short for 'endogenous morphine'). They are a form of natural pain relief, produced by the body to help us keep functioning when injured or stressed – during exercise, for example, lots of people report a 'runner's high', which is a feeling of wellbeing from the endorphin release. The production of endorphins in our system begins to rise during late pregnancy, and the increased levels of endorphins produced in a non-medicated labour have an effect similar to that of pethidine (*see* page 105), but without the side effects. In labour they also help us to zone out and enter a part of our brain where the overthinking and analysing of our frontal lobe (our 'executive brain') has no place. The levels of endorphins produced by the brain will be in direct response to the demand of the body for pain relief and so, if a woman has an epidural, the level of endorphins fall, meaning the baby gets less too.

An experienced home birth midwife will know that the reason women are less likely to ask for pain relief at home and seem to go into a trance-like state much more easily in this environment is because of the effect of endorphins and their uninterrupted production when labour is not being interfered with. So allow and welcome the flow of endorphins and don't question why you might be feeling slightly euphoric at times – just enjoy it!

Wonderful water

Following on from the subject of endorphins, one thing that helps to increase their production is negative ions, an abundance of which is found in turbulent water. They are thought to help us release endorphins and serotonin, both 'feel-good' hormones, which might explain why it feels so good to be close to a waterfall or standing near breaking surf.

Getting to a waterfall or the seaside in labour is probably not on everyone's agenda, but a good alternative is to stand under the flow of water from a 'power-shower'. Going into the shower, leaning your forehead against the wall and letting the water pound your lower back can do wonders for moving you on in labour. The subsequent release of endorphins will also help you enter 'the zone', enhanced by the sound of water literally drowning out other ambient sounds around you.

This can be a really helpful way of managing contractions. Showers are obviously available in birth centres and obstetric units too, but if it's your own shower and it's familiar and safe, that has an added bonus compared to using a shower that isn't yours. (Who was the last person to use it? Can I be sure it has been properly cleaned?)

Water can be used throughout the whole labour in different forms: you can start with deep warm baths to help with the tension, cramping and uncomfortable tightenings in the pre- or early labour phases; you can move on to using showers to help increase endorphins and to get you into 'the zone'; and, finally, once you are in really established labour (usually defined as at least 5cm, but generally I'd say hold off until you really feel like you need the use of water), climbing into a pool and allowing the warmth and depth of the water just to take you.

The key thing with the birthing pool is not getting in too early. It's an intervention, albeit a benign one, so if you climb into it too soon I think it can often switch off contractions after a while. Interestingly, this is not what the limited evidence says, but anecdotally I've seen it happen so many times over the years, I find it hard not to believe this is the case, perhaps because you simply get too relaxed.[22]

Climbing into a deep warm pool of water in the challenging last stages, the final transition where you are having very strong contractions, perhaps reaching what feels like the edge of your ability to cope, in these circumstances with the next contraction there might be a sweeping sense of relief and renewed belief that 'I can do this'.

If you're far enough on and there's a wave of relaxation that comes with getting into the deep warm water, it can often help the cervix dilate fully and can initiate the fetal ejection reflex, speeding up the last moments of birth through a strong release of oxytocin, endorphins and catecholamines. Women will often climb into the water, have that 'ahhhh, that feels so good' moment and then, particularly if they're having their second baby, get a sudden surge of energy, start to feel pushy and have a baby in their arms in no time at all.

There is another good reason to use a pool, which is not so relevant if you are having a home birth, but worth being aware of: women are out of reach from too much interference from their caregivers. When you're in a deep pool, your partner might climb in with you but it's very unlikely that your midwife or your doctor will. So you can isolate yourself rather conveniently by climbing into a pool – that's less of an issue if you know and trust you caregiver – but worth bearing in mind.

Transcutaneous electric nerve stimulation (TENS)

TENS machines are small, battery-operated devices with sticky pads, which you apply to your back.

How they work:

- Transcutaneous – through the skin.
- Electrical – TENS machines deliver small electrical pulses to the body via electrodes placed on the skin. TENS machines are thought to affect the way pain signals are sent to the brain.
- Nerve – pain signals reach the brain via nerves and the spinal cord.
- Stimulation – if pain signals can be blocked by the tiny electrical shocks from the TENS machine, the brain will receive fewer signals from the source of the pain.

There is little hard evidence as to how well TENS machine work as pain relievers, although one theory is that they can help stimulate your body to make more endorphins. Some women respond positively to using TENS and say that it really helped them through their labour, while others quickly decide they don't like the sensations at all and take the device straight off.

You can either buy them outright or hire them for a reasonable amount, so it's not the end of the world if you try it and it doesn't work for you. TENS is recommended for the early stage of labour in particular, but you might find it works for you all the way through. You must remember to take the pads off before getting into your birth pool though!

Entonox®(gas and air)

Another way of maximising the value of your breath is to combine long, slow breaths in with the use of Entonox®, otherwise known as gas and air. It's a mix of 50 per cent oxygen and 50 per cent nitrous oxide, an analgesic that you inhale through a mouthpiece to provide a mildly sedative, calming effect – it won't block out the intensity of a contraction completely. Many women find it can really help them get through the more challenging stage of labour by enabling them to refocus on the breath. Your midwife will bring it with her when she comes out to you in labour.

As a contraction starts you begin a long slow intake of the gas, breathing it out slowly and evenly through the mouthpiece before taking the second breath. You continue in this way until the peak of the contraction, after which I will gently remind a woman to have a break from it. The effect will usually last the length of the contraction and then you can pause, breathe normally and be ready to start again. Although Entonox doesn't stay in the system, continuous use of it over a long period can make you feel woozy and a little 'out of it', so in my experience it works best if intake is focused on the first half of the contraction and then allowed to dissipate through the second half as the contraction ebbs away.

Don't be immediately put off if on the first try you are left feeling a little dizzy and/or nauseous. This is quite a common response initially, but it doesn't usually last and the benefits overall can outweigh the side effects if you persist. I have seen Entonox® work really well through transition, for example, when the rhythm of the contractions can get lost temporarily and you might start to feel a little overwhelmed and panicky. The messages you are receiving can get a bit confused at this stage in the labour because the direction of energy needs to begin to change: the upward energy that has been opening up the cervix begins to morph into the downward energy needed to push your baby down the birth canal ready for birth.

This change in direction sends mixed messages to your brain. I often think that is the real sign of transition, when women start to lose the plot a little bit and they're not quite sure what the messages are that they're receiving – and with that, they begin to lose the nice rhythmic breathing they have been using to cope with the contractions.

If this happens to you, using Entonox at this point can really help because it enables you to focus on each breath, using the mouthpiece to steady yourself, and, with the gentle encouragement and steady support of your birth partners, to get back into some sort of rhythm. At this stage I will try to be very tuned in to what is happening for the woman I am supporting ... it is almost impossible for her to articulate her internal sensations, especially from within 'the zone', but a slight panicky look in the eyes or a sudden need to move, to try to escape this feeling of being overwhelmed, is a common response to this intense period. If your caregivers are attuned to this and give you extra reassurance (it is okay, it is normal, you are doing great and you just need to focus on this moment/breath) and encourage you to breathe deeply to increase the amount of Entonox® in your system, you can get through this phase … and before you know it, you will begin to feel a little pushy as you move into the second stage.

If you know you would like to try Entonox, or you've used it very successfully in a previous labour, it's worth asking your midwives to bring plenty of supplies – you can get through a significant amount depending on when you start using it and ideally you don't want it to suddenly run out just when you are in transition.

Once you are seriously pushing, continuing to use Entonox can be counter productive and I might suggest trying one or two contractions without so that you can focus on and start to recognise the expulsive nature of your contractions and work with those rather than confusing the picture by still trying to breathe to a different and often unrelated rhythm.

Opiates

Options for opiate drugs to use at home are limited and should be used with some caution. The most commonly used one is pethidine and less frequently diamorphine. There will be some variation in what is available, depending on who is providing your care. They are known collectively as 'parental opioids', and although they do provide some pain relief for some women, the evidence is not clear and there are adverse side effects, including nausea, vomiting and drowsiness.[23]

There is also a potential effect on the baby, especially if the birth occurs shortly after the drug has been administered. In this case, the midwife will need to carry another drug to give to the baby if he or she is affected, to counteract the problem.

As you can probably deduce, I am not a great fan of these forms of pain relief at a home birth although I have seen them used to really good effect when there is a long latent phase with a baby in an unhelpful position and an already exhausted mother.

If you are interested to explore the option of using an opioid at your home birth, even if just to have it on standby, discuss the pros and cons with your midwife during your pregnancy and make your decision well in advance so that any additional arrangements that might be needed to access the particular drug can be made.

Possible Complications and Reasons for Transfer

I f you watch any drama on TV that involves one of the characters going into labour or having a baby, it will invariably be portrayed as an impending disaster that is only narrowly avoided by an emergency dash into hospital where heroic doctors save the day.

This is not only a very unhelpful depiction of imagined events, bolstering the idea that childbirth is inherently dangerous, it is also highly misleading because, in terms of transfers from a planned home birth, such 'life or death' emergencies are very rare (as evidenced in the Birthplace study (2011),[24] and now the latest national guidance from NICE, 2014).[25]

That is not to say that there isn't a need sometimes for speed and prompt action at a planned home birth, but the occasions when it is because of a genuine emergency are very few and far between. It is important to keep a proper perspective on the likelihood of a complication occurring at home when you are healthy, with a well-grown baby and a straightforward, normal pregnancy to date.

The other point to remember when thinking about the complications that can occur at a home birth or what the reasons for transfer might be, is that all midwives have regular and comprehensive training and updates about what to do in a variety of situations that they may face, wherever they work. There are often bespoke courses run for 'out of hospital' situations as well as increased opportunities for joint training with other specialties such as ambulance crew and obstetric colleagues to maximise good working relationships and seamless care. Midwives have annual updates, known as 'skills drills' or 'mandatory training', on all the main reasons for needing to take emergency action and so, should a need arise at home, your midwives will be well practised at responding appropriately and efficiently and will bring all the equipment they need for first response actions, such as resuscitation equipment and drugs to control any excessive bleeding. Although not a requirement in law, most providers aim to have two midwives present at the time of birth, with the second one being called as the labour progresses towards second stage. This is so that, should it be necessary, there are two pairs of hands available as well as it being a very supportive way of working. When I worked in independent practice with my midwifery partners Tina and Teresa, we knew each other so well that communication was honed to a look between us, or one of us would start thinking something just as the other said it out loud – continuity works for midwives as well as for women!

The possibility of needing to transfer, because of a problem for yourself or your baby does increase, however, when either of you have additional risk factors and/or you have been advised to have your baby in an obstetric unit. The decision is ultimately yours to make, but you will want to research your options thoroughly and ideally talk through all the potential risks and benefits with your midwife and obstetrician before making your choice.

This chapter is not designed to explore those situations in any great depth, however, as it is beyond the scope of this book to consider all the factors you will need to take into account if you are planning a home birth when you have additional risk factors or complications. 'Safety' is about far more than just the physical aspects of care and so you need to apply the advice you are being given to your own, individual and personal circumstances, and seek support and advocacy from those clinicians who offer it and whose opinion you trust.

Deciding to transfer

In my experience, making the actual decision to transfer is usually pretty clear and unambiguous. There comes a point, which is perhaps recognised and reached more easily where there are established relationships between everyone and a previous discussion has taken place, when the circumstances are right to move and everyone knows it.

Having said that, it's very important for you not to feel harassed or bullied into making the decision before you are ready. Acknowledging the (sometimes profound) disappointment of not achieving what might be the cherished dream of a home birth is crucial, as is revisiting the decision afterwards and processing it, ideally with the midwives who were there but, if that isn't possible, midwives from that team or hospital. Reviewing the circumstances of the transfer, especially with your maternity notes to refer to, and sometimes several times over, can help you to come to terms with the reasons for it if, with hindsight, you are not completely sure what they were.

One of the things I always make a point of saying during early discussions about the possibility of transfer and again, if there is time, during the decision-making process itself, is that once the moment has passed and you are looking back with the knowledge of hindsight, don't start beating yourself up for making the decision, even if you feel the need to have a clearer understand of the reasons that led up to it.

Once you are pain free and feeling more normal again, it is very easy to forget the effect of your emotional and physical state at the time the decision was reached and start to feel disappointed with yourself for not having 'stuck it out' or for making the 'wrong' choice. You may feel that if only you'd been stronger, more determined, less tired or whatever, you could have stayed at home and perhaps everything would have worked out fine. While it is impossible to state with absolute certainty what would have happened, I always tell women that if the decision feels right at the time, it invariably is and there is very little to be gained by revisiting it. It is really important to keep reminding yourself that you arrived at that decision under different circumstances and that it felt right at the time.

One way of avoiding negative feelings is to have had lots of discussions during the pregnancy about the potential reasons for transfer and how comparatively common it is, especially with a first baby. The Birthplace study shows a transfer rate of over 40 per cent.[26] Although that means 50–60 per cent go on to have a successful home birth, 40 per cent is still a sizeable minority and expectations should be managed accordingly. There is no failure with transfer – an important part of the overall planning and my own philosophy is 'if in doubt then transfer'. It is always better to be at the end of a successful and positive birth experience, wherever it takes place, rather than wishing the transfer had taken place earlier. There is no shame in transferring for additional help; in fact, it is usually accompanied with a general sense of relief.

A positive birth experience isn't necessarily about achieving a candlelit water birth with soft music playing in the background; it is actually much more connected to whether or not you felt in control of your decision-making and were given the information and time to reach your own conclusions, and then supported in them. You should be able to look back and feel as positive about the emergency caesarean you needed – and be aware of all the reasons why that was the case – as you would have been about that candlelit water birth.

Being given the time to get your head around the change in circumstances, as well as being treated with respect, compassion and kindness are the important ingredients in any situation, and that includes decision-making around transfer. It is rare that there is no time at all and, if that is the case, it is usually pretty clear why.

Labour and birth can be unpredictable and challenging in many different ways. Remaining open-minded and aware that plans may need to change goes a long way in helping to come to terms with any change that does happen, whatever it is.

What is crucial is the importance of trust in your relationships with the midwives caring for you. If you suspect that you are being pushed into making a decision to transfer that is more about their agenda – perhaps to do with staffing issues or shift changes, for example – you need to question their reasons closely (or get your partner to if you are trying to stay in your 'zone') and remember that you have the final say – it is your decision and that must always be respected.

Having said that, if there is a strong sense of trust and partnership between you all, then, in my experience, there is usually consensus and the decision-making process is very straightforward. It is okay to feel disappointed, of course, but you should never be made to feel either that you have somehow 'failed' – should you be the one deciding that you need extra pain relief – or that you were transferred, against your real wishes, for external reasons that had little to do with your own situation.

Reasons for transfer

I have been involved in plenty of transfers over the years. The most common reason is for slow progress although the underlying cause for that slow progress may vary. We will have given it our best shot and usually tried lots of different strategies as part of our constantly re-evaluated plan of care, but there are times when the baby's position isn't great, no matter what we do – perhaps because of anatomical misalignment, but sometimes just because that's the way it is.

Eventually we will look at each other and know that a bit of help is needed, perhaps to make the contractions stronger to tuck the baby's head in or because the mother is tiring after a long and gruelling pre-labour, followed by hours of strong contractions that don't seem to be getting her anywhere.

If it is a baby in the back to back position (posterior), often the mother has constant back pain on top of the pain of contractions and that can be really hard to deal with, especially after many hours. A transfer for an epidural might allow her body to relax and let go of the tension that has built up, she can get some much needed rest while the contractions are brought back – usually with the help of syntocinon (synthetic oxytocin) – and she may then feel revived enough to carry on and still have a vaginal birth with no further interventions.

If transfer is being contemplated, there should be no sense of rush or panic. A conversation takes place and a plan is made, which might involve trying another strategy for 30 minutes or an hour, resting/eating something/having a bath/getting out of the pool if she has been in for a while as that can sometimes slow things down … any number of things can be put in place, but, in the end, it isn't sensible to just sit at home indefinitely. The key for me is to know when the plan needs to be changed and to transfer when everyone is in a good place, emotionally and physically – the mother, the baby, the midwife – not forgetting dad either! There is no point pushing a situation to its limits and then possibly having to transfer under much more stressful conditions.

Action stations

The plan is agreed by all concerned and, once the decision has been made, everyone swings into action. Usually the midwife will contact the hospital to alert them – this will normally be the hospital where the woman has already booked in as they will have her records and test results available, but occasionally it might be more sensible to just go to the nearest unit – it all depends on the circumstances.

The form of transport chosen – whether by ambulance or by private car – will depend on the circumstances. If the labour has stalled, for example, and nothing very much has been happening, it makes more sense to go in under your own steam, but again these are decisions that will be taken at the time, depending on the clinical circumstances. It might be that you have one or two midwives with you and that will also influence who does what and how the transfer is managed.

If there is an active clinical situation – any bleeding, or concerns about the fetal heart, for example, it is important to use an ambulance because if there are any further concerns on the journey, you are then in the right place to access additional help; plus, of course, an ambulance can switch on the blue light and get through early morning traffic much easier than you will be able to in your own car.

Sometimes, if the midwife is on her own and busy clinically, it makes sense for the woman's partner to make the call to the ambulance service, especially as they can give local details about the area and where to enter the building (if you live in a flat, for example). Some midwives, including myself, will carry a useful 'aide-memoire' of what the partner should say.

Usually I will suggest at the Birth Talk that it is always worth packing a small hospital bag with essentials in it, which can then be tucked away and forgotten about if it isn't needed – it is so much easier if you have already gathered everything together in one place instead of your often tired and possibly emotional partner trying to think through everything you and the baby might need, while also trying to help you get dressed and ready to go. If possible, I always try to clear away my equipment and do some tidying up (unless there is someone available to do it once we have left) as it is so much nicer not to come back to a mess after the birth!

Other children

The other thing to consider is any other children in the house (*see* pages 53–5). My own practice is always to have talked through the different options available to the family should the need to transfer arise and then get them to have a clear plan in place about who can be contacted in what circumstances. It is worth bearing in mind that transfers from a planned home birth for second or subsequent babies are much less common in all the research and evidence to date – more like 8–10 per cent according to the Birthplace study (2011)[27] – nevertheless it can and does happen and it will be very important to have a previously agreed plan that can then be seamlessly activated.

Perhaps a neighbour has been primed to come in if the children are asleep upstairs, or maybe a grandparent is already staying with you. If it is during the day and the children are at school there should be an arrangement in place for someone to collect them and have them for tea or a sleepover as appropriate.

In a real emergency, of course, if there was no one else available it might be that the father would need to stay with the children until reinforcements arrived to take over. In that case, the midwives would accompany you in the ambulance and your partner would follow on as soon as he could.

The journey itself

Where there is no rush and the journey itself can be calm and unhurried, I always travel with the mother and her partner in their car. I think it is better that we all stay together, and if she is using Entonox® I can help support her through her contractions, leaving her partner free to concentrate on traffic, directions etc., although ideally he will have done a practice run before the day itself to familiarise himself with where to park and where the entrance is etc. It is always worth having discussed all of this with your midwife beforehand. This is much easier if you know who is going to be with you, but even if it's a midwife whom you have never met, you can have written a birth/transfer plan and agree the details with her when she first arrives.

What is important is that all your caregivers remain calm and supportive of you during the preparation and the journey itself. Choose them with some care if you are having extra birth partners as the last thing you need, should a transfer become necessary, is to have to start taking care of them because they are having a meltdown. If you are using an ambulance, the crew will normally be wonderfully calm, patient and caring. This is a normal day to them and they will be keen to put you at your ease and reassure you that you will be well looked after.

What are the most common complications?

Please note that 'common' is used in the sense that these complications are the most likely ones to occur, not that they happen commonly. So let's look a little more closely at what the main reasons are for transfer – other than slow progress or the need for additional pain relief.

Fetal heart anomalies

When you are in the first stage of active labour, the NICE guidelines recommend listening in to your baby's heartbeat every 15 minutes for 1 minute immediately after the end of a contraction.[28] It is known as 'intermittent auscultation' – as opposed to continuous monitoring where you have two belts around your tummy picking up the fetal heart and the contractions. The latter is known as cardiotocography (CTG) and is never done at home. (Indeed, it shouldn't be offered in hospital if you have no additional risk factors as there is no evidence that it is any better at picking up potential problems.[29])

This recommendation of listening to the heart rate so frequently is not based on any evidence but on a consensus reached through negotiation. It will give the midwife a snapshot of how well the baby is coping with labour. If the heart rate is within the normal range of 110–150 beats per minute (bpm), there are no dips or 'decelerations' and there is a good variability (over five beats difference), it gives reassurance to the midwife – and actually to everyone in the room – and is written in your notes as part of the record of your labour.

If, when listening in, the midwife picks up any anomalies in your baby's heart rate, that will prompt her to observe more closely over a short period and may include her asking you to change position. These transient abnormalities usually resolve themselves very quickly and are probably due to temporary constriction or compression of the cord for some reason in utero. If, however, it is a long and non-reassuring 'bradycardia' (when the heart rate falls well below the normal level and doesn't come back up again), it may prompt her to make a quick decision to call an ambulance, even if only as a precaution in the first instance. She should always be prepared to immediately share her concerns with you, but in a calm and measured way since clear communication is key to good decision-making.

Sometimes, though, what might sound quite alarming to you is within the normal patterns of fetal heart rates at different stages in the labour. In second stage, for example, when you are actively pushing and your baby's head is being squeezed in the birth canal, it is very normal for the heart rate to drop temporarily as a result, but then to climb back up to normal rates as the contraction wears off and the head compression eases.

Your midwife will be trained in all aspects of recognising fetal heart rate compromises and her suggestions in response to any variations from the normal pattern will be affected by other factors, such as whether or not you are already fully dilated, if you have had a baby before and whether or not there is also meconium (baby's first poo) in the amniotic fluid if your membranes have ruptured.

Bleeding during labour

Women sometimes worry if they see blood when they are starting to go into labour or are beginning to get stronger contractions, but often it is just what we call a 'heavy show' – where the mucus plug that sits in your cervix throughout pregnancy has absorbed some blood from the tiny blood vessels in the cervix, which rupture as the cervix starts to soften and change. Bleeding during labour is known as 'intrapartum haemorrhage' (IPH). Even though the mucusy discharge that you might see on your pad or when you go to the loo can look alarmingly bloody sometimes, it is rarely a problem and is actually a good sign that the cervix is doing things. You can usually confirm this is what it is by checking that it has a 'sticky' quality to it – it is usually a little darker in colour, different to bright red, active bleeding. If you have the latter you need to get it checked with your midwife/hospital straightaway.

Sometimes you can have bleeding because part, or all, of your placenta detaches from the wall of the uterus. Known as abruption, it is usually linked to some specific risk factors, such as scar tissue from a previous caesarean or after surgery or treatment that occasionally might leave the lining of the uterus compromised or damaged in some way. Symptoms can vary and sometimes bleeding isn't always obvious externally, so you should always mention any unexplained abdominal pain in labour that continues after the end of the contraction.

Occasionally the cause of bleeding might be to do with the position of the placenta on the uterine wall. Placenta praevia, which is when all or part of the placenta is over the cervix, can sometimes remain undiagnosed in labour, even when you have had scans during the pregnancy. There is also the possibility of a ruptured uterus, although, without a previous history of surgery or other risk factors, this is rare. Your midwives will be alert to any unusual bleeding during the labour itself and will recommend immediate transfer if they have concerns.

Cord prolapse

Cord prolapse describes the situation where the umbilical cord drops down (prolapses) either alongside or below the baby's presenting part, which could be a head, bottom, shoulder, knee or foot. It can happen when your waters break or after they have already broken. It is a serious situation that requires swift diagnosis and immediate action on the part of your midwife to reduce the risk of a poor outcome.

It is important to note, however, that if you only have one baby onboard, you have reached full term (37–42 weeks pregnant) and you have a well-grown baby whose head is nicely tucked down into your pelvis, the chances of experiencing a cord prolapse are very low. The risk increases when your baby is breech (bottom down) or transverse (lying across your tummy) or when your baby is premature, when you are expecting twins or when you are being induced and your membranes are ruptured artificially or spontaneously while the baby's head is still high (not in the pelvis).

If the cord prolapses and your midwife confirms this diagnosis, she will immediately ring an ambulance, ask you to get into a knee–chest position on all fours or to lie on your side with a couple of pillows under your bottom. The aim of both of these positions is to tip the baby off the cord. Your midwife may consider filling your bladder with fluid as another way of keeping the head up high, and will usually insert her fingers into your vagina to lift the baby's head off the cervix and try to reduce any compression on the cord. The idea is to try to ensure that the cord continues to pulsate, maintaining the flow of oxygenated blood to your baby.

You will usually be transferred into hospital for an immediate emergency caesarean. If, however, this is not your first baby, you are fully dilated and starting the second stage, in the unlikely event that you experience a cord prolapse, your midwife may use her clinical judgement to facilitate the birth – either at home, en route to hospital or once you arrive there – and ask you to push the baby out. With a second or subsequent baby, this may only take one or two pushes.

Shoulder dystocia

Of all the emergencies that can occur during childbirth, shoulder dystocia (SD) is one of the most difficult to ascertain accurate numbers/incidence for. Rates vary from 0.2–3 per cent, which in part is because there are lots of definitions and a lack of consensus about which are 'true' SDs and what are just a temporary difficulty with the shoulders – perhaps as a result of problems caused by the position a woman is in and the actions of healthcare professionals at the time of the birth.[30]

Whatever the true rate, however, genuine SD is a very serious complication that can cause permanent injury or even death. There are certain antenatal risk factors that have been identified, such as maternal diabetes, abnormal pelvic anatomy and others. Your midwife will discuss with you what all of these potential indicators are and, as your pregnancy progresses, will be alert to the development of any causes for concern, especially in relation to the size of your baby.

The word 'dystocia' describes an abnormal, slow or difficult birth; an SD is when, after the baby's head is born, the shoulders don't rotate inside properly and get 'caught' on the symphysis pubis and/or the sacral promontory – the bony parts of your pelvis – so the baby's exit is impeded. Women who are obese or expecting a big baby are automatically considered to be at higher risk of having an SD, but, in fact, 40–60 per cent of births where SD has been reported are with babies weighing less than 4kg and 70–90 per cent of big or 'macrosomic' babies are born normally.[31] It is therefore an unpredictable event – even in the presence of some risk factors – which begs the question about what else might be going on.

In normal physiological birth, when the woman is usually upright, either kneeling or squatting or similar, the baby moves down through the pelvis and rotates as necessary to negotiate the passage down. After the head emerges, there is usually a pause, although not always – occasionally a baby will birth in one fluid movement and within one contraction! Normally though, the head is born with one contraction and then, during the gap before the next one, the midwife waits to see what we call 'restitution', which describes the head rotating back into its natural alignment with the rest of the body.

Once that has happened, the next contraction will normally see the rest of the baby born with the shoulders slipping under the bony part of your pelvis because the baby is now positioned correctly.

What can sometimes happen, though, and which I saw more than once as a student midwife, is that the midwife or doctor, keen to help the baby be born once their head is out, doesn't wait for restitution to happen and may start to put traction on the head. If, however, the shoulders and head are not realigned, this can have the unintended consequence of pulling the baby's shoulder on to the pubic bone where it then gets 'stuck'. Impatience and not paying attention to the physiological flow of birth has caused the problem and then the procedures and actions needed to undo the problem have to be called into play.

The other mistake made by healthcare professionals (in this case caused by the actions or directions of the clinician who is 'delivering' the baby) for SD (also known in this instance as 'bed dystocia') is to do with the position that the woman herself is in when in the second stage. Despite all the evidence, as well as the theoretical teaching in midwifery education, that gravity and upright positions are best for both mother and baby, I am amazed at how common it still is to find women ending up on a bed either on their backs or, just as bad, sitting on their coccyx to push their baby out.

If you are healthy with an average size baby and no antenatal risk factors for SD, being at home, being free to adopt different positions and being encouraged to do so as the second stage progresses all increase the likelihood that you will not have a problem.[32]

If you do run into difficulties, however, your midwife will be tuned into and closely observing progress to ensure the baby is maintaining momentum through your pelvis. If she has any concerns, or suspects SD, she will take certain actions that will be very familiar to her and which she will have practised regularly, the first one usually being to ask you to get into a 'McRoberts position', which she will explain or even demonstrate and which resolves the issue in about 40 per cent of cases. If it doesn't, she will then move on to a series of other actions, which she will explain as she goes. When midwives and other healthcare professionals have regular and frequent training updates on how to respond to this emergency, the risk of long-term injuries reduces dramatically.

Resuscitation of the baby

'What if my baby doesn't start breathing?' is, understandably, one of the most common concerns that comes up when parents are thinking through the pros and cons of a home birth. It is therefore worth spending a bit of time explaining the physiology behind the process of the baby leaving his or her watery home and taking their first lungful of air.

There are some important differences in a newborn baby's system at birth. These protect their vital organs and mean that a short delay in taking their first breath after birth does not necessarily cause major oxygen deprivation or have the same potentially catastrophic effect as it would do in an adult. A well-grown baby at full term has been well prepared to cope with labour and birth. As with all mammals, the heart, for example, is packed with glycogen (the body's stored fuel or energy), which enables it to provide ongoing and adequate circulation for quite some time in the face of any temporary delay in taking that first breath at birth.

While inside your womb, your baby 'practises' breathing movements, during which the fluid in the lungs is exchanged with amniotic fluid. In the last few weeks of pregnancy, the amount of this fluid starts to reduce as it is gradually reabsorbed, so that in labour the remaining vestiges can be largely squeezed out during the baby's passage through the birth canal. As the baby emerges into air, he or she is stimulated to take their first breath and the lungs will normally inflate like two small balloons. However, just like when you are trying to inflate a new balloon, the initial pressure required to inflate the lungs is greater than subsequent breaths need to be. Once breathing has been established, the effort required to inflate the lungs each time is quickly reduced and babies adapt remarkably swiftly to their new environment.

Resuscitation and early clamping of the umbilical cord

Back in 1985, at an antenatal appointment just before I had my first baby, Lucy, we were discussing the third stage and the delivery of the placenta when my obstetrician, Yehudi Gordon, said to me that one day everyone would wake up to the realisation that the current practice of clamping and cutting the cord immediately after the baby was born made no sense from a physiological perspective. He explained that by doing so we were depriving babies of approximately one-third of their total blood volume, which would normally transfer from the placenta via the umbilical cord during the first few moments of life. I wasn't a midwife then but what he said made sense to me at the time and his words have remained with me over the years and have influenced my practice as a midwife.

It has taken most of the 30 years in-between, but finally it seems that it is now generally accepted that immediate clamping of the cord at birth isn't a great idea. In the latest guidance for management of the third stage, delaying the clamping of the cord for a few minutes is now recommended to enable the fetal blood in the placenta to pulse through the cord and into your baby.

The new and more accurate phrase, 'optimal' cord clamping, to describe what is now being accepted as best practice is becoming more widespread because clamping the cord immediately at birth is actually 'early cord clamping' and therefore should not be advised unless for some reason the cord is not functioning at birth and the baby is in immediate need of active resuscitation.

The reason why this distinction is important, aside from the beneficial effects for the baby of avoiding hypovolaemia (low blood volume), is that, if for any reason your baby is born requiring any help to take his or her first breath, leaving the cord to pulsate ensures that the richly oxygenated blood from the placenta is continuing to flow into the baby and acts as Nature's back-up support system.

The act of clamping and cutting the cord and then whisking the baby off to be resuscitated at the other side of the room, away from the parents, is being rethought in many birthing units and there is now an alternative, developed by a doctor and known as a Bedside Assessment, Stabilisation and Initial Cardiorespiratory Support (BASICS) trolley. This trolley can be more easily brought to the baby, who can therefore remain attached to the cord and stay close to his or her mother if some help is required to get his or her breathing started or established.[33]

The chances of your baby needing a significant amount of help to start breathing after a normal labour and without any previous signs of fetal compromise are very small. Figures from a Swedish survey suggest that of low-risk babies beyond 32 weeks gestation and following a normal labour, about 2 per 1,000 needed resuscitation unexpectedly and, of those, 90 per cent were successfully resuscitated using a bag and mask (which is the equipment midwives use at a home birth in the United Kingdom); only 10 per cent of this number (i.e. 2 per 10,000) needed further treatment (intubating).[34]

When I am at a home birth, in common with most midwives, I will lay out and check all my supplies, including resuscitation equipment, ready for that unexpected event. The reality is that, with gentle stimulation, which is achieved through drying the baby with a warm towel as he or she is born and is being passed over to you, the vast majority of babies will take their first breath within the first minute or two and will often accompany it with a short period of crying to stimulate their lungs and clear any remaining fluid. A warm environment and drying the wet baby is very important in every birth as they lose heat very rapidly, but is especially important if a baby is unresponsive, and these actions need to be implemented immediately.

If additional help is then required, as midwives, we will all follow a very similar and well-rehearsed, step-by-step procedure, using the ABC approach:

- Checking the Airway is clear, especially in the presence of meconium (baby's first poo).
- Initiating Breathing as soon as possible, using a face mask attached to a pressure bag if necessary.

- Checking Circulation, starting chest compressions if the heart rate is below 60bpm and, as discussed, leaving the cord intact and pulsating.

The midwife will use exactly the same procedure as if you were in hospital, and everything will be done next to you, with an explanation being given as she works. She will be quick to call for extra help, sometimes asking your partner to ring for an ambulance – often as a precaution, as it is rarely needed – and, by the time the crew arrive the baby is invariably pink, warm and enjoying skin to skin time with you.

Bleeding after the birth and/or placenta delivery

As we've discussed throughout this book, one of the potentially scarier elements of planning a home birth can be thinking about the 'what ifs'. Perhaps the most common 'what if' is being worried about whether you might lose too much blood after the baby or placenta is born – known as postpartum haemorrhage (PPH). The amount of blood loss that constitutes a haemorrhage may be defined as more than 500ml here in the United Kingdom, though in many countries it is 1 litre or more. Perhaps the most helpful way of defining a problematic haemorrhage is 'any amount of blood loss that compromises the woman's wellbeing'.

For many years the routine intervention, either immediately following the birth or with the birth of the baby's first shoulder, was for the midwife to inject an oxytocic drug into the woman's thigh, then clamp and cut the cord; then, within a few minutes, the midwife would aim to be actively delivering the placenta by 'guarding' the uterus and pulling firmly on the cord.

There was little debate about this practice: the evidence showed that overall there was a lower blood loss for the mother with an 'actively managed' third stage and that it was therefore safer for her than a physiological third stage that used no drugs and relied on maternal effort to push the placenta out, usually in a longer time frame.

There is now a wider debate and a better understanding about the benefits of a natural, or physiological third stage, including the element of optimal cord clamping and the adverse effects associated with having certain drugs to control the amount of bleeding. There is also a greater recognition of the pregnant woman's physiological ability to cope with a higher blood loss around birth because she has an increased blood volume by the end of pregnancy of around 40–50 per cent more than normal.[35]

A woman choosing to have a home birth may also have a preference for a physiological third stage if it is in line with her overall aim to have as little intervention as possible. Whether this is the case or not, all midwives attending a home birth will carry a range of drugs to control and manage the amount of bleeding after the birth and will usually have ascertained what your preference is and talked through the circumstances under which they would recommend giving you the injection.

Immediately after the baby is born, during those first lovely moments when you are meeting your baby for the first time, your midwife will be quietly observing and monitoring blood loss. If you are in the pool, she may ask you to come out if for any reason she is finding it hard to monitor the quantity, but usually her check will be very unobtrusive.

As with all the other regularly rehearsed 'skills drills' for potential emergencies, at home or in hospital, midwives are well used to acting quickly and decisively if they have any concerns about your bleeding, either before or after the placenta (although it is while the placenta is still in situ that the greatest attention is paid to any constant trickling or gushes of blood). Women vary considerably in how they are coping with blood loss and, if you are feeling at all lightheaded or unwell, you should always let your midwife know and she will investigate further.

Once the placenta has been delivered, it is carefully checked to ensure it is complete and, if your midwife has any concern that it is not, she will talk you through some options, which may or may not involve transfer, depending on your individual circumstances.

Although the most common reasons for excessive bleeding are to do with the placenta – either its position or that it has only partially come away from the uterine wall – bleeding could also be caused by tears or lacerations to your cervix or vagina, a tear or rupture in the uterus or if your uterus is atonic (i.e. too relaxed), which is more likely if it has been contracting for many hours and has run out of energy. Again, your midwife will be aware of all of these possibilities and will be checking continuously that all is well and bleeding is within normal limits.

Pre-eclampsia/eclampsia

If you have had regular antenatal appointments throughout your pregnancy, you will be well used to having your blood pressure checked and your urine tested at each one. These two elements, especially if combined with excessive swelling (oedema) are monitored because they are commonly, but by no means consistently, associated with the condition known as pre-eclampsia (a condition in pregnancy usually diagnosed by the presence of high blood pressure and a large amount of protein in the urine).

The incidence of this condition in its milder form is thought to be 5–10 per cent in the United Kingdom, and 1–2 per cent of cases will be very severe.[36] There are some common risk factors associated with pre-eclampsia that your midwife will have talked to you about (usually at booking) and any signs of it developing after 20 weeks of pregnancy will be followed up at your antenatal checks.

This means that you are unlikely to have got to term and be going into labour without any idea you may be at risk of developing pre-eclampsia. However, if your blood pressure does start to rise rapidly in labour or you complain of visual disturbances, severe pain under your ribs or a sudden severe headache, your midwife will consider transfer. This is because of the risk of eclampsia (fitting or convulsions), which, left untreated, can lead to you or your baby becoming very ill.

Last word

There is always an element of risk with any undertaking in life, and the journey that is labour and birth, wherever it takes place, is no exception. Of the potential difficulties that may occur at a home birth, many come about because of a unique combination of circumstances that may occur at an individual level but are not easily defined or quantified. We also know from the evidence that they are not common.[37]

When an unexpected event does occur, however, midwives are highly trained, competent and skilled practitioners who will invariably be very efficient at dealing with any problem that arises. It is always a good idea, as part of your preparation and decision-making, to have a conversation during your pregnancy, ideally with the midwife who will be with you in labour, about what you might expect from the normal procedures and guidelines for home birth of the hospital or care provider you are booked with, and about details such as average transfer times during labour.

In the end, you need to weigh up the pros and cons of what you feel comfortable with in terms of the different choices you can make. What feels like an unacceptable risk of being out of hospital for one woman will be outweighed by the strong instinctive need to be in a safe, known space for another. That is both the joy and challenge of actively choosing a home birth – in the end it is entirely an individual choice, which only you – and your partner – can make.

Prolonged Pregnancy and Going 'Postdates'

Medical induction means starting labour intentionally with the use of certain drugs. There are a whole host of reasons why it might be advised, some of which are because of a medical condition or concern that has developed during your pregnancy. In these situations the advice is that it is safer for the baby to be born sooner rather than later and examples include high blood pressure, pre-eclampsia (*see* page 131) and obstetric cholestasis (a potentially serious liver disorder). There are other, non-medical reasons such as 'advanced' maternal age (over 40) where the advice nowadays is to induce earlier. However, prolonged pregnancy – going past your due date – is still the most common reason for offering women a medical 'elective' induction of labour.

Normal length of pregnancy

There are a number of different answers to the question of how long pregnancy lasts, depending on how you calculate it and when you ovulated. For thousands of years women have used the phases of the moon to calculate their menstrual cycle and, when their period doesn't happen, they suspect they are pregnant. A lunar cycle is just over 29 days, which adds up to a gestational period of 290 days or ten lunar months.

Your 'due date' is based on a calculation that was first proposed back in the 1700s. It assumes you have a 28-day cycle lasting from the start of one period to the start of the next and that you ovulate exactly in the middle, i.e. at 14 days. It is known as Naegele's rule[38] and is based on historical rather than observational data. The formula that will give you the expected date of birth (EDB) is to take the first day of your last menstrual period (LMP), subtract three months from it and then add one week. Interestingly, if you were to use the last day of your period instead of the first, the date would be similar to the lunar cycle calculation.

Example:

First day of LMP is 12 November
12 November minus 3 months = 12 August
12 August plus 7 days = EDB 19 August
12 November to 19 August = 40 weeks

The problem with Naegele's rule is that it is based on your menstrual period, not on ovulation. The reality, of course, is that every woman has her own individual cycle and for some women it may be longer or shorter than the average of 28 days. Ovulation usually occurs 14–15 days before the first day of bleeding, so the due date will be later for women with long cycles and earlier for those whose cycles are shorter. But it is also possible to ovulate towards the beginning or the end of your cycle, not necessarily bang in the middle.

There has also been some recent research on the length of pregnancy, which suggests a variation of as many as 37 days from the date of conception (not menstrual period),which is one more reason why it is helpful to describe a five-week period, from 37 to 42 weeks, when your baby is 'term' and could arrive anytime.[39] The researchers also calculated that only 4 per cent of women birth when predicted and only 70 per cent within 10 days of their EDB, and so having a specific time span of 40 weeks isn't actually very helpful.

Ultrasound is now the preferred method of determining your 'due date' in the United Kingdom. Various measurements of the baby are taken and number-crunched by computer software to give you the EDB. This may differ, sometimes markedly, from the date worked out from your LMP or even when you know for sure that you conceived. Once we add in Holly Dunsworth's new theory about the trigger for labour being the limits of our own personal metabolic load (see page 203),[40] then the argument for pinning the arrival of your baby on to one day becomes increasingly absurd.

So, to return to the question about the length of the average pregnancy, you can be pretty sure that no one can give you a definitive answer, whatever they say! If we aren't sure about that, how can we know when pregnancy is prolonged or postdates?

Non-medical ways to get labour started

There are many different suggestions and ideas about how you might encourage labour to start spontaneously. While there isn't much research around the effectiveness of different methods, which include acupuncture, reflexology, using herbs and homeopathy, it can feel positive to take action yourself if you feel the clock is ticking towards an induction date. I would therefore advise you to do some research on the different options to decide which, if any, you feel comfortable with.

Membrane sweeping

This is one of the options that will probably be offered to you by your midwife, sometimes from as early as 39 weeks but more usually once you get past your due date. There is some evidence that it is effective for bringing on labour but that it can cause discomfort and minor bleeding.[41] Some women are keen to try anything and everything to avoid the induction route; others prefer to just wait and see if/when labour starts spontaneously. It is entirely your choice.

DIY suggestions for encouraging labour

Diet:

- Pineapple contains an enzyme that helps to stimulate hormone release.
- There is some evidence that eating six dates daily for the final four weeks of pregnancy can be helpful

Sex:

- Having sex, especially with orgasm, releases hormones associated with the onset of labour. Sperm is rich in prostaglandins; nipple stimulation releases oxytocin. Making love is a really good way to get in the mood for labour to start!

Clary sage oil (use with caution and advice from a qualified aromatherapist):

- Sniff clary sage drops on a tissue – you can put this under your bra strap.
- Put 6–8 drops in the bath – ideally, have a bath a day.
- Burn it in an oil-burner.
- Use it for massage. Mix 6 drops of clary sage oil with 1 teaspoon of base oil (keeps for 24 hours).

Ankle acupressure:

1. Dip your forefinger in the oil mixture.
2. Find acupressure point SP6. This is located on the inner leg, four finger widths up from the ankle, in the groove under the bone.
3. Circle your oiled finger in small circles, using medium pressure – this shouldn't hurt – for 5 minutes on each leg. Take care your finger does not slide away from the pressure point.
4. Repeat three times daily.

Tummy massage:

1. Use the clary sage oil mixture to very lightly circle your fingers around your abdomen, with one hand following the other hand, and making sure one hand is always in contact with your tummy.
2. Cover your tummy with a warm towel, and just lie and relax.

Walking:

- Go for a walk outside for ideally 30–60 minutes a day. Try to include some uphill and downhill walking.
- Spend time walking up and down the stairs slowly. Aim for 30 times up and down, with every other step taken

sideways. Make sure to use both sides. Pause with one foot up on the next step (or two steps up) and rock and circle your hips. Repeat at least twice a day.

- Include deep squatting twice a day, for at least 5 minutes, to help your baby descend into your pelvis.

Induction of labour

Many hospitals now agree a date for induction that is either just before or at 42 weeks. Although this is a little later than it used to be, it is still a big deal for most women, even those who are planning a hospital birth, and for those who planned to have a home birth, it can be quite devastating. There is some very interesting language used around 'going postdates', or 'over your due date', with lots of women assuming that they aren't 'allowed' to go beyond 42 weeks (as if somehow they have now surrendered the right to make that decision for themselves, just by reaching a certain date or stage of pregnancy).

So the first thing you need to be really clear about is that any decision to be induced is yours to make and you can choose not to accept the hospital's offer of induction if you prefer to wait to go into labour spontaneously. The national guidelines on this subject give you different options, which your midwife and doctor should discuss with you if you get to that stage.[42]

You can either choose to accept what is being offered, or negotiate a different date for your induction, or decide to do neither and choose 'expectant' management, which simply means waiting for labour to start naturally but with the offer of regular monitoring while you do so. This usually involves a scan to measure the volume or depth of amniotic fluid around the baby, to check the blood flow through the cord and to assess how healthy your placenta looks.

You can also go into the day assessment unit in your local hospital every few days to have continuous monitoring (CTG) for half an hour or so to check the heart rate of your baby. In addition, you will be asked to be aware of the frequency of movement from your baby.

The evidence used to recommend induction of labour beyond a certain date concludes that the stillbirth rate begins to increase slightly from 41 weeks and goes up further from 42 weeks onwards.[43] It starts from a low base though so your risk goes from 2 to 3 per 1,000 to 4 to 7 per 1,000. Some have argued that, if your baby is well grown and you have no other risk factors, your actual risk of having an unexplained stillbirth is as low as 2 per 1,000.[44] The challenge, of course, is how you weigh up for yourself the risks of going over 42 weeks versus the risks of induction itself.

There is other literature that analyses some of the randomised control trials and looks at the evidence around routine induction.[45] If you feel strongly that you really don't want to be induced, it is important that you have a good read through all the evidence that exists so that you can try to reach a decision that feels right for you.

Revising your choices after 42 weeks

If you do get to 42+ weeks and you are offered an induction date that you decide to go ahead with, it is really worth having a discussion with your midwife and doctor about whether or not they use Propess (a 24-hour slow release prostaglandin inserted into your vagina). Some Hospital Trusts are happy for certain women to go home overnight to await contractions and so there may be a conversation to be had about whether that is an option open to you. There is also a logical next question, which you may or may not wish to explore: if, upon your return to the labour ward you are contracting regularly, your cervix is dilating, the pessary is removed, your baby's heart rate is fine and you don't require any other intervention, can you go home to continue labour and, providing all continues to be well, birth your baby there as per your original plan? Chances are the answer will be 'no' until there's more data giving reassurances about home-based inductions, but it's perfectly possible to envisage this scenario as a reasonable option in the future.

The Immediate
Postnatal Period

I'm not going to go into a great deal of detail about the postnatal period or establishing breastfeeding (if that is going
to be how you choose to feed your baby). There is already plenty
of information and advice out there, in books and online, which
you can pick and choose your way through, or not, depending
on your preferences.

However, I do want to flag the importance of honouring
this special time. I suggest two key principles, which I hope will
chime with your own thoughts about this period as an natural
extension to your home birth.

If you have just had a successful home birth that you have
planned and prepared for, chances are you will be on a
wonderful oxytocic and endorphin high. Even if it is just
relief that you feel initially, there are some lovely hormones
flooding your system for the next few days, especially if you
do lots of skin to skin and encourage your baby to be at the
breast as much as possible. So this is a time for really closing
the front door against the world for a few days and spending
some 'quality time' with your new baby and closest family –
enjoying your babymoon!

First key principle: (I include this in my Birth Talk with all
the women I care for.) Spend a week 'in bed' (well, not literally

the *whole* time – you can potter around your bedroom!) and a week on the sofa. We seem to have lost the idea that a woman who has just given birth needs time to recover, and stories abound of new mums nipping out to the shops on Day 3 or entertaining a houseful of visitors when all she really wants to do is go to sleep.

The importance of resting – being nurtured, pampered and supplied with nutritionally delicious food – cannot be stressed enough in my view. The huge advantage you have after a home birth is that you don't need to get dressed and come out of hospital. You can have a lovely bath or shower after a home birth, then climb into your own bed and just stay there! The reason why this is so important is that after the birth it's not unusual to feel like you could climb Everest. You might then be tempted to be up doing lots of things, wasting this precious energy, so that when you start to come down off the high and in all likelihood the effects of sleep deprivation are beginning to kick in, you will have no reserves; *also*, once you add in the hormonal surge that arrives around Day 3 with the milk coming in, you may come crashing down – known as the 'baby blues'. On the other hand, if you stay in bed, conserve your reserves, eat really well and sleep when your baby sleeps, you will be much more likely to coast down nice and gently.

Second key principle: If you want to breastfeed, please remember that what you do in the early days is crucial to establishing your future milk supply. Ensuring wherever possible that your baby has his or her first feed within the first hour of birth is a really great start – but only a start. Many babies will then have a well-deserved sleep lasting a few hours, after which they should be encouraged to wake and feed again as often as possible and at least every three hours.

Sometimes, a baby will be sleepy and disinterested in the breast in the first day or so, although this is much less common in an unmedicated birth. If this is the case with your baby, you should hand-express the colostrum (the yellowish fluid, rich in protein and antibodies, that is present just before and a few days after birth) just as frequently and give it to your baby via a syringe or on a teaspoon to make sure they remain well hydrated. On the second or third night, be prepared for a mammoth feed. It may start around 10.00 or 11.00pm and continue on and off until the early hours. If you know that this can happen and that it is normal and very common – I usually describe it as the baby 'calling' the milk in – hopefully you won't start worrying that it might mean you don't have 'enough' milk. In preparation I would suggest that you try to get a good stretch of sleep the day before!

If you keep in mind that all the baby really needs for the first couple of weeks or so is sleep, food and cuddles, with a few nappy changes thrown in, it might help you manage these first days without putting too much stress on yourself to 'get it right' – instead, remember that it's almost impossible to 'get it wrong'!

PART 2

Birth Stories

How the birth stories were born

When you're considering the pros and cons of a home birth, other women's experiences can be invaluable in helping you make the decision that's right for you. You might hear birth stories by talking to people you know, attending a local home birth group, watching videos online or reading. Although there are plenty of them 'out there', I wanted to include a selection of stories in this book to complement the rest of the information.

Some of these experiences are from past clients of mine, and others arrived in response to a request I made on social media during the writing process in 2015. I asked for recent experiences from women and their partners around the country – ideally in the last 12–18 months – so I hope you will find a set of circumstances here that you can relate to. Some women (and men) chose to send answers to the questionnaire I sent out, while others preferred to write in a narrative way. I have included a mixture of both.

I am hugely grateful to everyone who participated – I know how busy life is with small babies/toddlers!

The stories are mostly quite different, but in my opinion there is a common thread: they all illustrate, in one way or another, the transformative power of birth and the sense of 'ownership' that is conveyed through the lived experience of choosing to birth your baby at home.

Second baby after poor experience with firstborn

Caroline Weighton

My overriding memory of my firstborn's birth was not the calm water birth or lovely birth midwife, but the 7am paediatrician's visit the following morning. The staff flicked on all the fluorescent lights (it was still dark in late September) and announced that the doctors were doing their rounds. Most of the babies had been taking it in turns to cry throughout the night, so most of us were only just settled. I was there as a first-time mum, on my own, and had not been able to stand up since giving birth without fainting. All I wanted to do was go home, be in my own bed and have a shower in my own bathroom.

When thinking about having another baby, a home birth was always in the back of my mind. So when asked by my community midwife at my booking in appointment if I would consider it, I answered yes. My husband, however, took a little persuasion – largely because of the amount of 'mess' it might create! As we talked more about it and got advice from a friend who happens to be a very experienced midwife with home births, we both became comfortable in the knowledge that this was the birth experience we wanted. One practical argument was that I would rather plan for the birth to happen at home than for it to happen there unexpectedly, due to a speedy labour or being snowed in during December when I was due.

We researched what we would need. I wanted a water birth again, but we would need to find a way of fitting this into our maisonette. We found a mini inflatable birth pool that would fit in our lounge and could be blown up fairly quickly. It had plenty of space for me and took less water than some of the other pools we looked at. My husband got stuck into organising all the equipment (sheets, towels, waterproof sheet for the bed, pool accessories) and found himself with a level of responsibility that he hadn't had when we were in hospital for our daughter's birth.

My contractions started at 4.45am on 24 November 2014. They progressed fairly steadily and by 8.30am I was kneeling over my birthing ball, swaying around. My two-year-old daughter came and hugged me, wondering what on earth I was doing. She seemed slightly unnerved, but the childminder soon came to pick her up. I then rang the labour line, a central coordination point for North Hants women in labour, to let them know I was in the early stages. They made the on-call midwife aware and told me she would be in touch. As contractions progressed, I rang them again, asking for a midwife assessment as they had advised me to do. The assessment showed that I was 3–4cm dilated. I was told that once things got stronger, the midwife would come back and 'settle in' for the birth. Our midwife friend was also in a position to come to the delivery, so she arrived shortly after we made the call for the midwives to return. My husband set up the pool and then I felt the soothing relief of the water as I climbed in … and there I stayed for most of the afternoon and evening! I remember the contractions being much gentler than with my daughter, but the whole thing was dragging on and on.

At around 7pm I felt slight discomfort in my back and we all decided an examination would be a good idea. I moved out of the pool and lay on the bed. The midwife discovered, as she suspected, that baby had turned back to back and was wedged in my pelvis trying to come out face first. I didn't feel worried by this and felt quite safe knowing I was in experienced hands. I changed position so I was on all fours with my head on the bed to try and get baby to drop out of my pelvis. The midwives went into another room to call the labour line to tell them they were going to try and turn the baby. When our friend came back to do this, she felt that baby had already moved and then my waters broke. I have never experienced this before and it felt like there was a huge amount of water that just kept coming!

Our baby then decided that it was time to get moving and with nine minutes of pushing, and with me having managed to get back in the pool, he arrived at 9.54pm. My husband helped me scoop him up and our little boy screamed his lungs out! He was covered in vernix as he was 10 days early and had a bit of a bruised face from being stuck – no wonder he was so vocal when he came out.

We sat quietly in the pool looking at our brand new son in the low evening light, waiting for the cord to stop pulsing before cutting it and then waiting for the placenta to deliver. I came out of the pool to lie on our sofa, giving our son his first feed while the midwives checked me and then him before swaddling him up warm for his dad to hold. I got to wash in my own bathroom (although we had to boil water in a kettle as we had used up all the hot water for the pool!) and got tucked up in my own bed.

My husband and the midwives tidied and he had the pool down, cleaned and towels in the washing machine before coming to bed at around 1am. I lay in bed with snores either side of me that night, but knew that I was not on my own and was comfortable that no one else was disturbing us … I so enjoyed the moment. Our daughter came home the next morning after having had a fun sleepover. She looked at her new baby brother with excitement, saying 'baby' and seeming very pleased with the new addition to our family.

The whole experience was much more relaxed and calm than my first birth and enabled us to immediately bond together as a family in the comfort of our home. I felt much more 'normal' after the birth as well, which may have been due to it being the second time around but also because I didn't have to experience a more medicalised environment. I have now shared my experience with several friends who are opting for home births, hopefully showing that it is a positive experience for all involved.

A father's perspective

Magnus Weighton

How/when did you make the decision to have a home birth?

My wife first had the idea of having a home birth. This was based on the poor experience she had in hospital after the birth of our first child. She wasn't in a comfortable place, she and our firstborn, Elin, were woken throughout the night, and she didn't reap any rewards from that stay, such as superb help with breastfeeding or great advice. It wasn't my choice to have a home birth.

What was the reaction/response from healthcare professionals?

We have a friend who is a home birth advocate and midwife, who was understandably supportive. Other healthcare professionals were also supportive. Alton's healthcare professionals seem to have quite a positive attitude to home birthing.

What was the reaction/response from family (including your partner)?

I'll answer this question from the partner perspective. I was initially sceptical, having concerns that being in hospital was the closest that you could be to the best care. However, I was easily swung towards supporting my wife's decision as our friend is a midwife who supports home birth and she gave us a lot more information about it. I was concerned that we are quite a way from the nearest hospital, but our midwife said the travelling time from our home to the hospital was only eight minutes, which allayed that worry. The main reason I bought in to the idea was the idea of giving birth and then just going to bed!

I had some concerns about what I should be doing in the run-up to the birth, and during the birth itself. As a very organised person, I wanted to make sure that I had done everything I needed to do, but there didn't seem to be a written plan anywhere for what guys need to accomplish. In the end it was all well prepped and went pretty smoothly.

What was the reaction/response from your friends and wider circle of acquaintances?

Friends were a little surprised when we told them that we would be having a home birth but were very respectful. After the birth it's exciting to look back on the fact that it took place at home, and it can become a talking point.

Thinking back, what was the overall experience like? Did it meet/surpass your expectations (or perhaps it wasn't what you expected at all, e.g. because you had to transfer or it was more/less challenging than you were anticipating etc.)?

I believe it was more or less what I was expecting, perhaps surpassing expectations. This was in spite of the birth having a slight complication in that baby was stuck back to back for some time. However, once the midwife realised this, it was quickly remedied and things moved on speedily after that. It was a revelation to wake up with our new family the next day in our own bed! We were very lucky in that we had our fantastic pro-home birth friend and midwife there through the entire birth. Remember that with home birth you will get a dedicated midwife *and* a second midwife for the birth – a definite plus!

Using your own experience, what would your advice be to someone thinking about having a home birth?

Think about the risks from a couple of angles: firstly, whether there's a strong risk of complications during birthing that would necessitate a trip to hospital. Secondly, if it's a second child, consider whether the first labour was very quick. If so, it's likely that the second child will be quicker and a home birth may be inevitable. Consider the use of a pool at home. It's not too messy and does help relieve stress during birthing. If using a pool, then do think about how you will fill and top it up with hot water, and how you will clean it all away afterwards. Also consider using a waterproof bed sheet over your existing bed sheet, with a throwaway set on top. When all is done, you'll be able to whip the top layers off and have a fresh set already on the bed! Remember to stock up on snacking foods, even though you're at home, and have water to sip throughout.

Despite increasing evidence that, for many women, home birth is at least as safe as hospital with very good outcomes, the national home birth rate is still only around 2 per cent. What do you think needs to change to enable more women to make this choice/make this option more accessible and mainstream?

Health visitors, midwives, GPs and associated professionals need to buy in to spreading the message. This will only
be achieved if they realise WHY home birth is a safe and
appropriate option. Only then will they confidently pass on
the option to expectant parents, who will be able to weigh
up the options.

Hypnobirthing and water birth at home

Valerie Farndon

Early on in my pregnancy my midwife asked me if I would consider giving birth at our local midwife-led unit. I said I thought hospital would be best. I was sure I'd need intervention with my firstborn, like all the other women in my family. A few months later, and completely by accident, I ended up on a private hypnobirthing course with my husband. After the first session I realised that a home birth was what I needed. I didn't want to be worrying about when to leave home or if there would be a pool available. I didn't want my husband to have to go home on his own afterwards. I suddenly understood how important it was for me to be relaxed and in control of my environment. My husband and midwives were very supportive of my choice – without their support I would never have had the courage.

Many people believe that birth is a process that requires medical help, that it is hugely painful and that women can't do it on their own. Consequently, why would anyone do it at home without support and intervention? Our hypnobirthing course taught us that this doesn't have to be the case – women are designed to give birth and doctors often make things worse.

Unfortunately, our families didn't agree with us about home birth. My mother-in-law was a midwife in the 1970s and she was fully in favour of hospital births, intervention where necessary, and putting your chin on your chest and pushing. There I was, talking about dimmed lights, birthing pools and breathing my baby out as opposed to pushing it. She thought I was crazy. My own mother was also convinced that the women in our family didn't have pelvises designed for childbirth. Others in our family and friendship group all had the same reaction: that for your first baby you should give birth with doctors nearby. Eventually, we told everyone, apart from close friends, that we had opted for the midwife-led unit as a compromise.

My husband and I spent a long time preparing for the labour and birth. We practised our relaxation exercises religiously, we organised the pool, the music, even the snacks for the midwives. We knew exactly how we wanted the labour to pan out, and I spent a lot of time visualising how it would all happen. I think the planning and preparation really helped our birth progress. I would therefore recommend anyone planning a home birth to do similar amounts of research and preparation.

At 41 weeks the contractions finally began. They were sporadic, speeding up at night time so I couldn't sleep and slowing down during the day. Finally, after two nights of little sleep I had a membrane sweep that got things moving. There was a period of about half an hour, when I had to walk up and down the stairs sideways, as the midwife was concerned that the baby's head was not properly in position. After that, though, I spent the rest of the time in the pool. I drank lots of milk to keep my energy levels up, snoozed when my body relaxed, and breathed through the contractions with my husband's help. Throughout the whole process the baby's heartbeat and mine remained the same, never speeding up, never slowing down. Everything happened as I expected and hoped, it was hard work but I never doubted that we would get to the end successfully.

I strongly believe that if I had been in hospital, I would not have managed the birth I wanted. I was exhausted when I finally went into established labour, but being able to remain where I was, feeling comfortable and not having any other distractions meant I stayed stress-free and was able to focus solely on what my body was doing. I also had the opportunity to move around to help the head get in the correct position. I am certain that the reason my birth went to plan was because it was planned to be at home.

Elsa was born shortly after midnight. I hadn't needed any pain relief, and I didn't need any stitches. Around three o'clock our midwife tucked us all up in bed, ready to greet our first morning as a little family. I felt ecstatic for weeks and months afterwards, I had achieved the birth of my dreams. Some people said that we had been 'lucky'. In some respects we had, but our birth did not happen by chance.

I'm not really sure about what needs to change to make more women feel confident about choosing a home birth. I think that most women probably don't have a realistic grasp of 'risk' and are not aware of the statistics. I also think that women need to start seeing birth as a natural process as opposed to something that requires medical assistance. So many women I know say that they need to be in hospital in case something goes wrong, but my belief is that being in hospital is more likely to cause things to go wrong.

Second baby born before arrival of the midwife

Sarah Mullen

Just by way of some background, I've been married to Joe for five years. I had my first daughter, Nieve, at the age of 30 in July 2012 and my second daughter Zoe at the age of 32 in August 2014. We live in Wokingham.

How/when did you make the decision to have a home birth?

I'd always wanted a home birth as I was born at home, but when pregnant with my first child I knew that my husband wasn't comfortable with the idea. I believe both birth partners need to feel comfortable with the birth plan, so we opted for a hospital birth. I planned a water birth on the midwife-led unit at the Royal Berkshire Hospital (RBH) but I went 13 days overdue and my labour was induced. It was a quick labour (3 hours 18 minutes) but very intense and I felt like my labour was very medicalised – I was monitored in the delivery suite, was constantly on gas and air, and almost had a forceps delivery. As soon as I found out I was pregnant again, I spoke with my husband and midwife about my strong desire to have a home birth as I was keen to have a much more 'natural' labour in the familiar surroundings of my own home.

What was the reaction/response from healthcare professionals, your partner, family, friends and wider circle of acquaintances?

When I told my GP that I planned to have a home birth, he responded: 'Why on earth would you want to do that?' Then, more gallingly, he added: 'What does your husband think about all this?' Luckily, both my husband and my community midwife were really supportive, as were my family, given that my Mum had two home births herself (when that was even rarer than it is now). I also have two friends who had home births so they were informative and supportive, and I joined a home birth support group to draw on the experience of other local mums.

Thinking back, what was the overall experience like? Did it meet/surpass your expectations (or perhaps it wasn't what you expected at all, e.g. because you had to transfer or it was more/less challenging than you were anticipating etc.)?

In the end it felt like I had a home birth by default. I started to have very small twinges of labour pain at 2am. By 3.15am my contractions were five minutes apart, so we started to fill the pool. I called my parents to come and look after my two-year-old and I put in a call to the RBH labour triage line. At this point, I was told that they were short-staffed, had closed the midwife-led unit and I couldn't have a home birth. My husband wanted us to set out our rights and push for a home birth but I was reticent about doing this and so agreed to go into RBH.

I'd been using hypnobirthing CDs throughout my pregnancy and, as we got into the car, I put on the track aimed at helping you cope with an unexpected change in circumstances. My contractions spread out to every 7–9 minutes as I think my body reacted to this change. I was examined by a midwife at 5am, who told me, to my surprise, I was only 1cm dilated and my cervix had not yet softened. She told us to go home and wait until my contractions were three in ten minutes before calling. She said that the day shift would come on at 8am so we'd be more likely to have our home birth after that time. I didn't want to go home at this point as by now I'd psyched myself up for another hospital birth. I told the midwife about my quick previous labour, but she was pretty dismissive and again advised me to go home.

We arrived home just before 6am with my contractions still every 7–9 minutes apart and not overly painful – I felt I could manage them with my hypnobirthing techniques. I got into the pool at 6.40am, thinking to myself it may be too early as you're supposed to wait until you are 4cm dilated. I felt the initial soothing power of warm water when I first got in but after a couple of minutes I had a really powerful contraction and turned to my husband and said 'I can't do this without drugs' – yes, I was in transition! He had just dialled the triage line to ask if we could go back in when I shouted, 'I need to push!' It was clear to all that things had progressed really quickly and I wouldn't have time to get back to hospital, so an ambulance was scrambled and the on-call midwives alerted.

It was at this point that I started to panic. Giving birth without a midwife present was certainly not part of the plan and my hypnobirthing went out of the window. I begged for my Mum to come and join my husband and together they hauled me out of the pool and on to all fours on the dining room floor. My waters broke and the urge to push was overwhelming. The ambulance call-handler stayed on the line and directed my husband to tell me to just go with my body and push if I needed to push. By now I was hyperventilating and screaming, which upset my two-year-old, who came running into the room. Thankfully, my Dad was able to take her out for a walk. The paramedics arrived after 18 minutes (that felt like a lifetime to me) and my daughter, Zoe, was delivered a few minutes later at 7.30am weighing 3.1kg (7lb 3oz). She had the cord loosely wrapped around her neck, which the paramedics dealt with quickly. The midwives arrived about 15 minutes after she was born (40 minutes after we had called triage) and took over from the paramedics at that point.

I can't fault the care I was given by the midwives once they were there, but I was sorely disappointed not to have had their support and direction through the pushing stage. I believe it would have been a much calmer, quieter birth had a midwife been with me as I wouldn't have felt so panicked. Fortunately, my husband and Mum were so unflustered and supportive that I think they would have coped fine had the paramedics not made it either. I also firmly believe that even if I had planned a hospital birth, I would have given birth at home anyway due to how quickly my labour progressed, so at least I had everything around me for a home birth rather than trying to scramble together old towels and waterproofs at the last minute. It wasn't the calm, uncomplicated home birth I had envisioned, but once Zoe was safely in my arms I was so incredibly grateful to be in my own home and to be able to have a shower and then climb into my own bed with my new baby within a couple of hours of giving birth.

Using your own experience, what would your advice be to someone thinking about having a home birth?

Research home births and other labour options to make sure you and your birth partner are both really comfortable with this as your preferred option. Seek out the support and experience of others who have had home births so you can fully prepare yourself logistically and mentally. If you have other children, plan ahead for their childcare during your labour and birth – I would have preferred for my daughter not to see me in the pushing phase as I think it distressed both of us. I also wish I had been assertive in demanding a midwife the first time we called the triage line.

Despite increasing evidence that, for many women, home birth is at least as safe as hospital with very good outcomes, the national home birth rate is still only around 2 per cent. What do you think needs to change to enable more women to make this choice/make this option more accessible and mainstream?

All healthcare professionals need to be better at supporting it – my first touch point with the NHS was that initial appointment with my GP, who practically ridiculed the idea. Had I been less strong willed, I may have backed out at that point. The NHS needs to ensure that all staff work in line with its recommendations. They also need to ensure that there are dedicated home birth midwife teams, completely separate from the hospital teams, so women in labour aren't denied a home birth at the last minute.

Traumatic first birth; home birth with continuity for second baby

Holly Donoghue

I gave birth to my first daughter in hospital (NHS) and was left absolutely traumatised. Thinking about it almost three years on still fills me with dread. I knew that if I was lucky enough to fall pregnant a second time, I'd have to do things differently.

After researching my options carefully, I decided that an independent midwife would fit the bill perfectly. I'd have all of my antenatal appointments at home, support during labour and more comprehensive postnatal care than I had first time around. I'd book into a different hospital, and armed with my own midwife things would be much better.

A home birth had not occurred to me until the question was raised during my first appointment. We discussed the idea and I was told I could decide at any point during my pregnancy. I loved having this power of choice. 'Choice' was something that did not seem possible first time around. I was never given options, just guided down a path that I assumed was the only route.

With Annie and Sharon, my Neighbourhood Midwives, I received amazing support and invaluable advice from the start. I looked forward to my appointments and loved having the continuity of seeing the same face each time. This filled me with so much confidence that the thought of a home birth began to excite me.

When I informed friends and family of my intentions, responses ranged from being totally unfazed to politely horrified. It interested me that it was my own age group (early thirties) who showed the most concern. Older friends and relatives had a much more relaxed 'good for you' attitude. My husband and Mum, who had both been present the last time, were all for it.

It was during my pregnancy that NICE began to issue statements about home births being better for mothers and as safe as hospital births for babies. I felt this gave me a good foundation for my home birth argument when discussing the subject, and actually when people 'pooh-poohed' the idea, it just made me more determined to make it happen.

My biggest desire was to experience childbirth as naturally as possible. Rather than being on another planet through sleep deprivation and drugs, too exhausted to push and subject to a forceps delivery, I really wanted to 'feel' the experience as I imagined it should be. I liked the thought that gas and air would be my only artificial pain relief and that I'd need to call upon my inner strength to get me through this. I wanted to see what I was capable of . . . and now I know.

Rather than just ticking boxes at each appointment, I was constantly learning and discovering new things about pregnancy and labour. It became obvious to me that most of the complications I'd experienced during my first labour could have been avoided had I been more informed.

Three months on, thinking about that day just puts the biggest smile on my face. It was THE most surreal thing I've ever experienced. Deep down I thought there was a strong possibility that I'd freak out and want to go into hospital once I went into labour, but the reality was quite the opposite. I was so relaxed, had so much trust and faith in Annie that I cruised through my waters breaking and early contractions without any anxiety. When she and Sharon arrived, everything progressed smoothly and, luckily for me, quite quickly. Breathing, a hot shower and quiet words of encouragement were all I needed to bring my second daughter into the world. Before I knew it, I was bathed and in my own bed with my new little bundle.

Looking back, the whole experience completely surpassed any expectations I had. To be given so much time and care by the midwives was absolutely brilliant. This is what I really missed out on during and after my first pregnancy. The wonderful postnatal care made a massive difference. Instead of muddling through the first weeks with a new baby running on caffeine, I was reminded to eat well and, most importantly, to rest. It sounds so simple but unless someone tells you ...

It was back to earth with a bump when I needed to get my baby ready for her newborn check within 48 hours of birth (on a Friday) and my GP refused to do a home visit. I was left feeling like a bit of a special and awkward case that they really couldn't assist. On the basis that I didn't feel like trekking down to the surgery in the first precious hours, we forked out for a private GP to do the job.

I understand that the government would like to see a rise in the national home birth rate – it's cheaper, after all, but without the necessary support in place I really can't see this happening. Although home birth is available, it was never offered to me. It almost feels like a 'special request', which may be fulfilled if you're lucky. I know one mum whose home birth wasn't possible at the last moment due to 'staffing issues'. Clocking on and off really isn't ideal and, in my opinion, a rise in caseload midwifery would be truly wonderful and make a massive difference to women.

Although I would recommend a home birth without hesitation, I would be reluctant to do so on the NHS, given the lack of support available. Obviously, an independent midwife comes at a cost, but as far as I'm concerned it's some of the best money you'll ever spend. Let's hope one day that this level of care is available to every woman. It absolutely should be – having a baby is a big deal!

First birth preterm and traumatic; second baby home birth with continuity

Sally Thompson

Edie came to me in a dream before I knew I was pregnant. It was one of the most amazingly vivid dreams I have ever had. In the dream I was giving birth, completely consumed by powerful waves of energy and joy. I pushed hard and out emerged my dark-haired daughter. I picked her up and held her close, she was warm and wet and slippery and I was ecstatically happy.

I woke from the dream in a sweat and disorientated. It was unsettling, as the previous few weeks I had been coming round to the idea that perhaps I wouldn't have another child and had even started getting rid of baby things. I had been thinking that after my first pregnancy and birth, which had been difficult and traumatic, plus two subsequent miscarriages, that perhaps we shouldn't push our luck any further. I felt we had been lucky with our son, who was born two months premature and had had a close call, and that the miscarriages might be a sign that we should stop. I was losing my nerve and afraid to get pregnant again in case something went wrong ... another miscarriage, or another difficult pregnancy or premature baby and all the stress that that had entailed.

Little did I know that the dream was actually a premoni-
tion, and also a powerful symbol of an experience I yearned
for. About a week after the dream, I realised I was pregnant,
and had mixed emotions, but the overriding emotion was fear.
Fear of my first pregnancy's problems resurfacing. And fear of
giving birth in a hospital and feeling so vulnerable again.

Together, my husband and I decided that we would do
all we could to mitigate the risks, even if it meant making
some financial sacrifices. I rested and took extra-special care
of myself. We asked my Mum to help look after our son,
so that I could rest enough, and also because by the second
trimester in my first pregnancy I had been almost bedridden
with back and hip pain.

I started researching the best ways to ensure a safer more
natural birth and avoid prematurity, and this led me to look
into independent midwives. After my pre- and postnatal
experiences in the hospital system the first time, I was thoroughly disillusioned with the medicalised bureaucracy that
had surrounded my son's birth.

While I was very grateful for the emergency life-saving
care that he received in the neonatal ward, I felt that the
surrounding pre- and postnatal care had been extremely
alienating and emotionally damaging to both of us as it was
so stressful, unnatural and unsympathetic to the emotional
and spiritual needs of mother and child. I really wanted a
different experience this time around and the best possible
chance for us to have a gentle natural birth, ideally at home.
From research I knew that the best chance for this was very
high quality, one-to-one midwifery care throughout the
journey, as well as a home birth, if possible.

I was really scared of ending up in hospital again and being bullied and ignored, which had been the case the first time. If something did happen that meant we'd have to have a hospital birth, I felt it important to have a midwife with me who could protect my space and wishes as much as possible.

And so after much research, we found and hired Neighbourhood Midwives early on in the pregnancy and I was fortunate to have two most wonderful midwives. I was lucky enough to have Annie as my primary midwife. She is serene, intuitive, warm and wise and an inspiration to the women she works with.

The pregnancy wasn't easy, I had lots of hip pain and my mobility was quite quickly affected. By the fifth month I wasn't able to walk much, but it was easier than the first time and I grew increasingly confident of having a positive birth experience. I also had the loving support of my husband and mother, and my friend, Kate, who herself has had two home births and is a pre- and postnatal yoga teacher.

I meditated on my dream often, it was as if Edie had sent me a message, saying, 'Don't worry Mama, we're going to be just fine', and I repeated positive affirmations or mantras daily and did lots of gentle yoga. And so, at 40 weeks, on her due date exactly and with a full moon in the night sky, Edie decided it was time to come out and see the world.

The day before her birth (a Tuesday) I had a visit from Annie and we discussed a consultant appointment that I had been sent for the following week, which was intended as a induction discussion. I felt it was too hasty to have the discussion and didn't want to even go to it. I was feeling very defiant and didn't even want to consider an induction.

I had a nice relaxing evening then went to bed. I woke up at 2.30am with mild contractions, which very soon got stronger and faster. I didn't want to disturb anyone unnecessarily, so I waited half an hour before waking my husband, Clifton.

As soon as I got out of bed, the rushes increased in severity. I had a very loose bowel movement, at which point I think my waters broke too. I phoned Annie and Kate while on the toilet and sensed everything was going to happen fast from that point on. I got downstairs and went into the head down position, and hoped Annie would arrive before Edie did!

With hindsight, I wish I'd just woken my husband up earlier and not been so concerned about raising a false alarm. As the rushes grew in intensity I gave myself over to them. They were overwhelming surges through my body and required all my concentration just to keep breathing through them. I tried hard to use the yoga breath I'd practised but really by this point it was all instinctive. I just went into my own world. It was like being in the ocean, with huge waves coming towards me and I needed to concentrate to meet each wave with as much calm as I could. At no point do I remember being scared or in pain though; it was just very powerful and primal and took me very deep inside myself and my body. It was me and Edie now, doing this together. At times I repeated my mantras: 'Each breath brings us closer' and 'Relax and open'. But really I was beyond speech.

Annie arrived just as I was going into transition. She said very little, but her gentle intuitive touch was all I needed. I got very hot and the rushes were so intense I started to moan really loudly with each one. The noise was instinctive. It felt good and helped release the tension.

Kate arrived shortly after Annie. It felt wonderful to be surrounded by the people I most trusted, and I felt calm and safe and relaxed because of that. Kate and Clifton helped support me as I knelt and leaned forward on the sofa. Annie rubbed my back, hips and thighs, which really helped. Things then slowed down a bit and I started to get a bit tired. It was at this point I really wished I had the pool to get into. I think it would have helped relax me and helped with the tiredness as my legs were starting to shake, but unfortunately it wasn't ready yet.

Kate caught my eye and reminded me to relax and open, which helped. It was useful to open my eyes and it grounded me as they'd been closed most of the time. Annie had me walk to the toilet to try and wee. This worked really well as it allowed me to relax some of my muscles, which I'd been struggling to do. I sat on the toilet and Annie suggested I put my finger inside and feel for her head ... and wow ... it was amazing ... I felt her head ... it was so close and so exhilarating! All of a sudden, I had an enormous powerful surge of energy, let out a very primal scream and had a huge contraction. I knew my daughter was about to born. We went back into the lounge and I knelt again. I gave two or three really strong pushes and then I reached down and felt her head. With another big push she was out. I had a fleeting concern about tearing just before she crowned, which may have caused me to tense up. With hindsight, I think rubbing or touching my jaw would have helped, or panting or coughing as she emerged, but she came out so fast there wasn't time.

Edie was born a little after 6am on Wednesday 3 June 2015, after about three hours of intense labour. I looked down and saw our precious daughter, she let out a strong cry and I reached down to where Annie had caught her and I brought her up to my chest. Warm, wet, slippery and with dark hair ... just like my dream.

I held Edie close, and Annie made me comfortable on the floor, sitting on top of a bed pan, to rest while we waited for the third stage to begin. My daughter was perfect and extremely healthy and larger than we expected: 4.3kg (9lb 7oz)! I delivered the placenta easily after about 20 minutes. We checked the cord and placenta and made sure the cord was no longer pulsing before Kate cut it. Then Annie made me comfortable on the sofa and we relaxed a bit. Edie opened her eyes and looked straight into ours and then she latched straight on to feed.

We rested and had some tea. Everyone was on such a wonderful natural high. About an hour after the birth, Annie and Sharon examined Edie, and then Clifton finally got to have a proper cuddle with her. Annie and Sharon, my secondary midwife, checked my perineum, which had torn (just a first-degree skin tear but a fairly long one). I chose not to be sutured as I had read a lot about first-degree tears not needing suturing and Annie and I had discussed this previously. Fortunately, it has healed nicely after six weeks of careful rest.

Sharon and Annie stayed a few hours, making sure all was well and getting me safely and comfortably into bed. Those first few hours and days are so precious, and it was such a luxury to be so well treated and to be in my own home and bed. I was on a natural high for days afterwards and we could focus on just enjoying our daughter and bonding as a family. Ultimately, I believe it was a healing experience for all of us. Also, as a result, Edie is a much more relaxed baby and we have been able to settle into a happy rhythm quite quickly.

The postnatal care from Annie and Sharon was superb too. It made a huge difference to my postnatal recovery to have the continuity of care from such knowledgeable and empathetic midwives so – for me it was just as important as the one-to-one care during pregnancy.

Something I've learned on this journey is the importance of asking for help and not being too proud to accept it. Also, how crucial it is to be surrounded by people you love and trust, to believe in yourself and your innate ability to give birth naturally, and to trust your instincts, especially when bonding and caring for your newborn. It also makes a big difference to believe in yourself as a mother. Every woman's journey and each birth are so different, but ultimately it should feel empowering no matter how it unfolds. I needed to feel safe, loved and protected to achieve this, and fortunately I was surrounded by people who made it possible to have a beautiful birth experience.

A quick birth with hypnobirthing

Katy Redford-Traynor

Four weeks ago I had a home birth using only hypno-birthing. My baby's 18-year-old brother and close family were downstairs and they were amazed at the gentle noises instead of anticipated screams. My mother-in-law said it was a hugely emotional experience listening to her grand-child being born and hearing lovely noises as opposed to fearful sounds.

My husband was with me and our midwife only just made it on time as I was only two hours birthing. We birthed in our dimly lit bedroom as the pool was not filled quickly enough as the birth was so quick. It was very special and I loved every second of it. My five-year-old was woken up after the placenta was birthed and he did his special job of checking if we had a boy or a girl. He also cut the cord with Dad! It was a truly family experience and was so special.

A positive experience of continuity

Rebecca Burnett

How/when did you make the decision to have a home birth?

My Mum had a home birth with her second and third babies, so it was always something that I had thought about.

What was the reaction/response from healthcare professionals?

When I mentioned home birth, I wasn't initially given any information regarding it so I wasn't sure what to expect and how things would work at home.

What was the reaction/response from family (including your partner)?

My Mum and Dad were very supportive as they had had two home births themselves. My husband was a little worried at first due to the problems we had around the labour of our first son. His heart kept dipping, and it was nearly an emergency caesarean section. Some family members would say, 'That's what hospitals are for.'

What was the reaction/response from your friends and wider circle of acquaintances?

I tried not to tell too many people as they all decided to tell me their own birth story that went wrong and I didn't want to be put off.

Thinking back, what was the overall experience like? Did it meet/surpass your expectations (or perhaps it wasn't what you expected at all, e.g. because you had to transfer or it was more/less challenging than you were anticipating etc.)?

From start to finish the experience was amazing. I had control over where I wanted to sit/stand/walk in the house, and the comfort of my own home allowed me to feel very relaxed. The midwife was fantastic. She knew what my concerns were and what I wanted for my birth as she had previously carried out my antenatal checks. She allowed me to make my own decisions, while guiding me with her knowledge and expertise. The midwife set up and cleared away everything, allowing me to enjoy quality time with my son straightaway.

Using your own experience, what would your advice be to someone thinking about having a home birth?

Go for it! Try not to let others put you off. If it's what you want and you are allowed to deliver at home, make the most of it all.

Despite increasing evidence that, for many women, home birth is at least as safe as hospital with very good outcomes, the national home birth rate is still only around 2 per cent. What do you think needs to change to enable more women to make this choice/make this option more accessible and mainstream?

I think the community midwife situation should be reassessed. I was very lucky in that the same midwife who did all my antenatal checks was able to be there during my labour. I feel that building the relationship before birth is important so that mothers-to-be feel more at ease knowing who will be at their house delivering their baby.

Second baby at home after previous transfer

Eulalie Charland

In 2011 I gave birth to my first son, Amyas, with the wonderful support of Tina and Annie from Neighbourhood Midwives. When I finally got pregnant with my second baby, I knew I would have to rely on the care the NHS could provide. I worried that I was meeting a different person at each appointment, but Tina and Annie had made my first birth enough of a positive experience (despite ending up in hospital for the last 20 minutes) that I felt pretty confident I could do this.

Friends and family expressed concern at my plan to give birth at home with a four-year-old present. That was the least of my concerns as somehow I knew instinctively that my bright little man would take it in his stride.

My waters broke at 1.30am, exactly like the first time. Two hours later my husband called out the midwives, just in time for me to start pushing. I felt strong and inwardly kept talking to my baby – we were going through this together as a team. My husband later told me that for him too, the whole experience was completely different from the first hospital delivery. He held my hand and saw our son appear without interference.

Auden Thomas was born at 5.03am, just as the first light dawned in the sky. This time I got to hold him straightaway and an hour later we were both tucked up in bed with a cup of tea. It was at that moment that Amyas, fuzzy-haired and bleary-eyed, stuck his head through the bedroom door and, seeing the midwives, gave a cheery grin and bid them 'Good morning!' before spotting his little brother in my arms. Perfect!

Second baby at home in water

Jo Burton

As a midwife myself, I've experienced most of what birth has to offer – good and bad. When I was pregnant for the first time, there was no question of where I wanted to give birth ... at home! Working in the community, I had been privileged enough to be present at some of the most wonderful births, seen excellent communication between professionals when home was no longer the best place to be, and – most important of all – witnessed what a woman's body can achieve.

First time around, since I wasn't classed as 'low risk' (due to my raised body mass index), the trust requested that I have additional scans and a meeting with the supervisor of midwives and the consultant. All of them were honest about the 'risk' but incredibly supportive. My husband and I joined a fantastic home birth support group, and looked forward to being able to call my midwife to tell her it was time.

At 41 weeks and 4 days my waters broke. I had a check-up at the hospital (I offered to go in since it was 3am and it seemed silly to wake up a midwife when I was having no contractions). All was well, so we went home to wait for things to happen. I walked, rocked and bounced. I had acupuncture and reflexology.

Before my waters broke, I had days of Braxton Hicks, but now ... nothing. The next morning I went into hospital for augmentation, using prostaglandin gel to stimulate labour. A monitor was attached to my baby's scalp (she was positioned back to back), I was given an epidural and I had a labour ward birth. Although I hadn't wanted it to be this way, the surprising thing is that it was lovely! Hypnobirthing helped keep me very calm and open-minded and everyone on the labour ward team was very kind. My labour lasted 10 hours from the first contraction, 4 hours active labour, and I pushed for a mere 20 minutes – not bad for a first baby! She was 4.4kg (9lb 10oz).

Throughout my pregnancy people had been telling me how big my bump looked, joking about me having twins, and asking whether I was sure I wanted a home birth. Lo and behold – here was this 'big' baby, who I breathed out without any problems at all. The funniest thing a midwife said to me after the birth was 'Wow, she's big! Thank God you didn't have her at home.' All I could think was 'What a shame I didn't ... that was so easy!'

I couldn't wait to give birth again. It's a euphoria that just can't be explained. When I fell pregnant with baby number two, we planned another home birth. Again we met with the supervisor and the doctors, and attended hypnobirthing classes. This time, however, I kept having unexplained bleeding. Everyone was a bit more cautious, but I felt confident and my wonderful midwives were very encouraging. The jokes this time were not about how big the baby looked but whether a midwife would make it in time. This made me nervous, but my husband, Dan, had been prepped about what to do in case they didn't arrive for the birth and he wasn't worried at all.

I had a sweep on the Sunday (40 weeks and 3 days) and at 3am Monday morning I woke up with a contraction that threw me out of bed. Any worries I had about not being able to recognise natural labour were quickly dismissed. Within half an hour the contractions were so intense that I rang my midwife. I explained they were only every five minutes but bringing me to my knees. She said she would come but that the second midwife had the gas and air and if I felt that I needed it to get Dan to call her.

I got into the bath but the pain was unbearable, so Dan rang the second midwife. By the time they both arrived, the pain had settled down. I could easily talk during the contractions and we all had a cup of tea. As the sun came up and nothing had changed, I asked if I could be examined. I was 4cm dilated and in established labour. This was it. The contractions intensified immediately and I started on the gas and air. There are some fabulous pictures of me laughing!

I got into the pool around 10am. It was so soothing, with daylight coming in gently through the curtains and country music on the radio ... I was in heaven. The midwives stayed with me the whole time, holding my hand, massaging my back. There were no interruptions (as was common in my first birth). Just us. I called my Mum (who had been looking after my daughter overnight to let me get some rest) to tell her what was happening and asked her to bring my little girl home.

My waters broke at 12.45 and there was a change. I felt panicked and overwhelmed. My midwife gently took my hand and whispered to me. Instantly I felt calm again. I felt safe. My husband started preparing for birth, the pool was warmed, and he told the midwives it wouldn't be long.

He knew me, he trusted them and there was an intuition in the room that can't be described.

I gave birth to my gorgeous Elodie shortly after 1pm in the pool. My wonderful husband got in with us. That was really special. He would never have done that in a hospital. He was a part of it. It was quiet, we explored her and she us.

I changed my mind about birthing the placenta in the pool and we all moved into the living room. After everything had been sorted, I was helped upstairs and into bed. Dan followed up with Elodie and we all lay in bed together. Uninterrupted (again, nothing like it is in hospital). She weighed 4kg (8lb 13oz). She seemed tiny to us. The midwives let themselves out and shortly later my daughter arrived. She walked into the room, saw the baby on the bed and climbed in and cuddled her. It was the most magical moment. That's where we stayed ... uninterrupted.

Hypnobirthing second baby after traumatic first experience

Clemmie Telford

My first labour was so terrible that I honestly thought my son, Bertie, would be an only child. Induction, hyper-stimulation, lots of blood loss, followed by an hour of panic attacks ... not ideal.

Cut to 13 months later and I'm pregnant again. The initial thrill of seeing that line appear soon gives way to a feeling of 'S***, I've got to give birth again!'

I was determined to do things differently. After some obsessive googling, I came across hypnobirthing. What a stroke of luck. A total game changer.

Our course at London Hypnobirthing was just brilliant. It forced me and my husband to discuss our fears, as well as confirming that home birth was the way forward for us. After months doing breathing, visualising and general prep, I felt ready and even a bit excited about my baby's impending arrival.

That was until my due date came and went.

With every passing day my anxiety levels crept up. Flashbacks to being induced with my firstborn were haunting me. I was convinced I was heading down the same route. Plus, I'd had contractions on and off for days – it felt like my body was tricking me and it was driving me potty.

At 40^{+5} I sent Hollie, my hypnobirthing guru, a rambling email about having a bit of a breakdown – even questioning my ability to go into labour naturally. She replied telling me to let go of the anxiety, to trust my body. IT WOULD HAPPEN. She was right. The next day I had a sweep. Only in pregnancy are you so pleased to have someone stick their hand up you. Turns out I was already 3cm dilated – woo hoo!

My midwife wished me farewell. Deep down, I think we both know we would be seeing each other soon. And that night I went to bed with a sneaky suspicion it was 'game on'. But given the false starts and with the help of 'hypno' I decided to get some sleep.

At 3.30am I was woken by a surge. It was definitely happening. No panic, no fuss. Just a real sense of knowing what needed to be done. With son number one safely dispatched to my sister, I got into the groove of labour … which mainly meant being naked and eating Jaffa cakes. Oh, and the midwife arrived.

There was a palaver with the birth pool. My husband had done a dry run, but crucially not a wet run – turns out the fitting couldn't connect to our tap (funny in retrospect, not very Zen at the time).

Eventually it was sorted. Once in the water I was able to breathe through my surges. Don't get me wrong, it was hardcore. Exhausting. At the time I desperately wanted it to stop. But at no point did I feel worried or out of control. Instead I just focused on getting to the peak of the surge then down the other side … 'Breathe in calm, breath out tension.'

Candles, chilled music (and yet more Jaffa cakes), pool. All very lovely. But I was getting into a bit of a mental downward spiral – transition maybe – and found the darkness oppressive rather than safe.

My midwife suggested that I might benefit from a change of scene. Once upstairs, the bright coolness of the bathroom felt like a new chapter. No sooner had I taken a seat on the loo than I was hit by one almighty surge. Properly a case of 'my body taking control': I leapt up, grabbed my husband in a strangle-hold for support, and out came baby's head.

Then with the next surge Woodrow Victor Telford made his entrance into the world. He was born calmly and quietly with his waters intact or 'en caul'. Swiftly followed by my placenta, which conveniently went into the toilet.

The relief was immense. I hadn't been induced. I hadn't used a scrap of pain relief. I hadn't bled. Just a tiny tear that healed naturally. And I wasn't pregnant any more!! I felt like the luckiest person alive.

Me and my new dude headed to bed. And that's where we stayed for the rest of the day.

When people ask me about my labour, I say it was everything I wanted it to be. A wonderful, empowering experience that made me feel like Superwoman, plus it got rid of all the demons from Bertie's birth.

Even writing this now, I want to do it all again. There really is no greater feeling than lying in your own bed at home, eating pizza, with your four-hour-old baby snoozing beside you.

PART 3

The History and Politics Underpinning Modern Childbirth

A History of Birth

The birth of a human individual is a fascinating event that has always attracted the attention of artists, philosophers, priests, and scientists. The very fundamental process of birth can be looked at from as many angles as there are fields of human interest. We can study the mechanism of the birth process, paying attention to the size of the baby and the dimensions of the pelvis, pondering over the cause and significance of the internal rotation of the child; we can study the physiology of birth, looking for causes of the onset of labour and uterine contractility, of post-partum haemorrhage; we can study the emotions of the expectant parents, their feelings of pride and anxiety, their expectations of the newborn baby; we can speculate upon the sensations that the process of birth evokes in the unborn and the newborn baby; we can study the significance of social conditions on the birth process and the influence of the birth rate on social conditions; in short, birth—like death—belongs to the most fundamental and basic facts of life.

Kloosterman (1982)[46]

Given the world population and the rate at which it continues to grow, we have to conclude that the human species is spectacularly successful at procreation. The majority of women giving birth across the globe still do so without professional assistance or intervention. My belief is that we are physiologically perfectly designed to give birth, and we have evolved over the ages – both physically and psychologically, to continue to do so successfully.

Perhaps the most significant of the adaptations we have made as a species evolving over the millennia has been bipedalism. From the time we began to walk on two legs instead of four, and from ancient women living within hunter-gatherer communities to city-dwelling women today, in spite of the vast social, environmental and cultural differences that have taken place, our bodies have not fundamentally changed physiologically and giving birth has remained essentially the same process.

Being able to give birth has always been an integral part of a woman's genetic make-up, and the power of a birthing woman has been deeply respected over the years because it is inextricably entwined in the roots of humanity. In order to understand the process of birth today and how it is constructed and experienced, it is helpful to look at our evolutionary history, so that, as Wenda Trevathan puts it, we may 'embody our past and make it an object of study in order to learn from it'.[47]

From an anthropological perspective, exploring the physical, biological and genetic origins of birth gives us some insight into how our bodies adapted and changed physiologically, and how, as a result of that process, birth came to be viewed as a social and cultural act.

The Industrial Revolution brought major structural changes in society, which ultimately resulted in birth becoming increasingly medicalised – a change so profoundly embedded over time that for the past four decades this version of the birth process has been seen by many as the only option there is.

The elements that embody this approach (i.e. having the process of your labour measured and judged against a standardised 'one size fits all' that is dictated by strangers, and then allowing those strangers to handle and care for your baby in his or her first moments of life) have become normal practice; and the interventions that are routinely offered in labour wards across the developed world are seen as an inevitable part of this.

And so, in a book about home birth, it feels important to me to acknowledge and remember our entire evolutionary past when considering our connection and attitude to giving birth today. In a sense, women contain this 'history' within their bodies – it is their link to every woman who has gone before them and is something to celebrate and revere.

Our ancestry

Human's ancestors, the first primates, appeared on Earth around 70 million years ago. Initially tree dwellers, they took their first steps around 20 million years ago. Living their lives in the treetops, they laid the foundations for the first humans, as the primate brain became progressively larger due to increasing brain power and intelligence. Their increased ability to learn from experience and their capacity to observe and process information meant that they soon became the most adaptable of all mammals.

Over time, primates also adapted the mammalian reproduction system to suit their own needs. Most significantly, they evolved a 'unicornate uterus', which meant females would normally bear only one child at a time and required only one womb cavity (by contrast, many mammals have a Y-shaped, two-horned uterus). To begin with, primate birth was considerably different to the modern human birth mechanism and a lot less complex.

Due to the morphology of the pelvis, the infant would descend the birth canal with no rotation and emerge facing forward in the same direction as their mother, so she could easily scoop them up in her arms. For this reason, primate birth was generally unassisted, and the individual birthing primate female had total control and autonomy over her birth – choosing where to deliver her infant and what position to be in.

She could even decide when to deliver. Primates have rarely been observed giving birth in the wild, and primatologists believe this is because the females can actually stop contractions and halt labour when they are uncomfortable with their surroundings or feel unsafe. Ask any farmer caring for a mare in foal and they will recognise this phenomenon. It is also evident that when a woman moves from her known surroundings into the bright and sterile surroundings of a delivery suite, her contractions often fade away.

Anthropologists observed that the primate birth mechanism began to mutate out of biological necessity as primates' skulls very slowly began to increase in size compared to their body mass. This process (known as 'encephalisation') continued as primates evolved into humans. There were gradual changes in the way the fetus began to lie in the womb, i.e. by curling up into an oval shape as opposed to lying in the shape of a cylinder. This led to the uterus working more efficiently and taking on a more positive and active role during labour, since encephalisation meant that the uterus had to actively direct and rotate the fetus during labour to accommodate the skull.

Natural selection favoured this change as it made birth safer for newer, larger-skulled primates; and giving birth to fewer infants also meant a better quality of maternal care and a deepening of the mother–infant relationship. These developments continued as the larger-brained primates started to birth earlier in order to fit their babies through the birth canal. With the length of pregnancy reduced, physical development had to continue outside the womb, meaning that infants became far more dependent on their mothers in the first stage of life.

When viewed through the lens of biological natural selection, this development could in some ways be seen as a disadvantage as it meant that the quantity of offspring a mother primate could produce in her lifetime decreased. However, this was offset by the quality of the infant, with its larger brain and capacity for greater intelligence. Another advantage was the positive social and behavioural relationship between infant and mother that now had ample time and space to grow.

Homo sapiens and bipedalism

Over 12 million years, primates gradually evolved into the first Homo sapiens. It was approximately five million years ago that evolutionary selection began to favour the anatomical and behavioural changes that led to the onset of the key evolutionary process known as bipedalism – the ability to walk upright on two legs.

The cause of this new type of locomotion, which is unlike that of any other animal species, is a matter for speculation, but it is probably best explained by Darwin's theory of evolution. Another possible reason could be that changes in climate and habitat led to migration from jungle treetops to the savannah plains, and living at ground level favoured a more elevated eye position. Another theory is that there could have been a need to reduce the amount of skin exposed to the sun. Or perhaps it was to do with the freeing up of hands for more dexterity, the use of tools and hunting.

As someone who loves swimming, a particular favourite of mine is the 'aquatic ape theory', pioneered by the writer and anthropologist Elaine Morgan in her influential (and controversial) book *The Descent of Woman* (1972).[48] Frustrated by the prevailing male voice in the evolutionary debate, her aquatic ape hypothesis proposes that our ancestors spent a period of time adapting to a semi-aquatic existence after they were driven to the seashores as a result of too much competition for scarce resources in the trees. Morgan argues that our bodies are relatively hairless to make them streamlined for swimming and in common with some aquatic animals our larynx is situated in our throat rather than in our nasal cavity. And in relation to birth, the reason why being in water during labour feels instinctively right for some labouring women may be because that's where our female ancestors gave birth!

The effect that walking upright had on pelvis development also led to fundamental changes in the way birth occurred, and so a different birth mechanism had to evolve for the new Homo sapiens. Primates and other four-legged mammals have a wide base; their centre of gravity is near the ground, and their spine acts as a long bridge, firmly supporting the body's weight on four pillars. By comparison, walking on two legs presented new mechanical problems never experienced by mammals before.

The new direction of the spinal column meant there was a smaller base to support an entire body weight and there were radical changes required to the way the pelvis was structured.

In response to these changes, the birth canal was re-orientated in such a way that the modern baby now has to go through a set of rotations in order to pass through without complications, a process that had already begun with the pre-human primates. There came about a connection and compromise between the newly developed functions of walking, posture, support of the spine and the birth process, so that bipedalism would not prevent the safe exit of the fetus at birth.

Pelves of primates

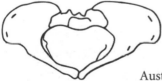
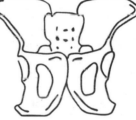
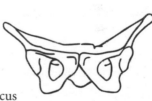
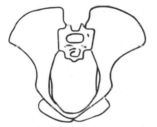
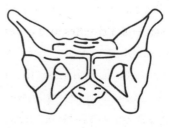
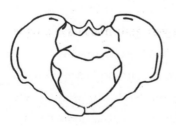

Pan

Australopithecus

Homo

The different types of female pelvis

After this initial big change to the fundamental design and function of the pelvis, which affected both men and women, pelvic morphology or restructuring continued for women and, over time, the female pelvis developed into four main pelvic types. Although similar in how they support the spine and operate in conjunction with the rest of the skeleton, there are considerable variations, which are affected by ethnicity, height, shape etc., but by far the most common type is the gynaecoid or classic female pelvis:

Gynaecoid: Classic pelvic shape, considered ideal for birth

Android: More masculine in shape and so narrower overall

Anthropoid: Usually found in taller women, and is wider front to back

Platypelloid: Wider side to side, with lots of internal space

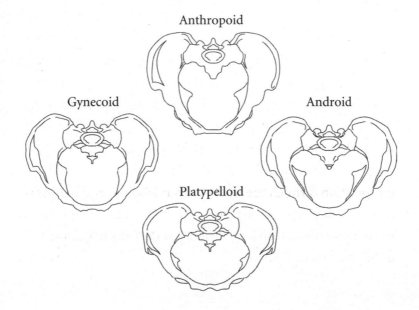

Anthropoid

Gynecoid

Android

Platypelloid

As midwives, we learn the different dimensions and meas-urements, from side to side and back to back, of each pelvis shape, as well as the dimensions of the fetal skull, in order to try to understand the relationship between the two and how it may impact on the labour process. A woman with a platypelloid pelvis, for example, can experience a long and challenging pre-labour phase, as the baby may take a while to engage and move down into the pelvis. But once that has been achieved, labour will tend to progress more quickly and be very straightforward.

It is helpful to be aware that a woman's pelvic shape may affect different stages of her labour, but what I've also learnt over the years is that the relationship between her pelvis dimensions and her baby's journey through it is an extremely fluid and flexible one. The different bony parts of the pelvis can move to accommodate the passing head, especially with the effect of pregnancy and birth hormones, and a woman is often very intuitive about what she needs to do to enable the process. This is why it is so important that you are free to be active and responsive to the sensations you experience during labour. In an instinctively active labour, during which you may move from all fours to squatting to lying on your side, the angles and capacity of the pelvis can change constantly, with the effect that your baby continues to move through it smoothly and without undue delay. If, however, you remain in one position through the whole of your labour – and in hospi-tal that often means being on a bed – it means the pelvis is much more static, with less capacity for the baby to exploit and utilise the available space.

The mechanism of normal labour – the labour 'dance'

It can be helpful to think about the process of the baby moving through the bony pelvis in terms of the three 'Ps': These are the Powers, or uterine contractions; the Passenger, or baby; and the Passage or pelvis (bony and soft tissue). The rotations the 'passenger' needs to make to come through the 'passage' are known as the cardinal movements of labour and consist of:

Engagement:	Baby first enters the pelvis
Descent:	Head moves down into the pelvis
Flexion:	Baby tucks head on to chin
Internal rotation:	Baby begins to turn mid-pelvis
Extension:	Baby extends head forward
External rotation:	Baby's shoulders rotate inside and the head realigns
Expulsion:	Rest of the baby is born

This process requires a constant readjusting and moving of the baby's head in relation to the bony pelvis, which is completely different to the obstetric mechanics of other primates. These minor readjustments are made by the baby, in tune with the mother; and, as I've explained earlier, the whole process tends to work best when you can be upright and actively responding to the sensations you feel. If you can 'dance' with your baby, the two of you working together, then it's far more likely to be an efficient rotational journey, which will maximise the 'power' of the contractions to ensure progress is maintained (*see* pages 80–81 for diagrams).

Why we need birth partners

These major structural changes in the pelvis, and the additional rotational aspects of the baby's journey, led to the most significant difference between primates and the first female humans. In the latter, because of the rotational element, the baby now emerges from the birth canal facing away from the mother. Interestingly, and perhaps as an unintended consequence, it began to prove more difficult for the mother, whatever her position, to easily reach down, as non-human primate mothers do, and clear a breathing passage for the infant or to remove the umbilical cord from around the neck. If a human mother tries to assist in her baby's delivery by guiding her baby from the birth canal, she risks pulling it against the body's angle, potentially causing damage to the infant or herself.[49]

So, going way back in time, the first Homo sapiens females began to realise they were struggling to manage birth on their own because of fundamental changes to their physical skeletal structure. The obvious solution was for a second person to be present at the birth – another pair of hands to safely catch and guide the infant into the mother's arms. Anthropologists believe this was the point in history when birth began to transform from a more isolated, individual activity to more of a social process, as more women began to seek assistance during their labours. The outcomes for these supported births, compared to managing birth alone, were more favourable, with the presence of another individual reducing the risk of mortality for both the mother and her baby.

It paved the way for heightened emotional states during birth, as labouring women sought help to guide them through their feelings of fear, anxiety, pain and vulnerability. This extra support also helped to meet the challenges of looking after infants with high levels of dependency when the mother was probably weary from pregnancy and labour and in need of some nurturing herself.

So began the very early stages of a transfer of 'authoritative knowledge'[50] from the birthing woman to her attendant, the earliest form of midwife, described by anthropologists as an 'obligate midwife'. Seeking assistance at birth was a uniquely human activity and gradually, over time, birth came to be seen not just as a physical process but as a social and cultural event with a host of ritual behaviours that would become deeply ingrained within each culture as time went on.

Thus, the transfer of the birth process into more of a social and emotional event was, in evolutionary terms, inevitable. With the advent of bipedalism, natural selection clearly favoured the option of assisted birth as it reduced the risk of mortality for both the infant and the mother. Therefore, current evidence, which confirms the value of having a known person at our side in labour, shouldn't come as any real surprise to an anthropologist. The reason why women desire supportive, familiar people around them at birth is because it's deeply rooted in our evolutionary history.

The helpless newborn

Along with bipedalism affecting the birth mechanism, there were other ongoing changes that were simultaneously having a significant impact on the birth process. Encephalisation, which began in the primate period, continued so that babies were being born with increasingly large heads compared to their body mass. The compromise here between the natural selection of larger brains, coupled with relatively narrow birth canals, was to move a substantial amount of brain growth to the post-natal period, which in turn led to babies being born in a state of 'secondary altriciality', another of the uniquely human elements of modern birth.

Put simply, secondary altriciality means that the baby is born in a state of helplessness and dependency and so will need everything to be done for them until their brain can 'catch up' in the development stakes. A newborn baby's brain is roughly one-third of the size of an adult's, but the rate of brain development in the first year of life is quite extraordinary, growing to more than two-thirds of its adult size in that short period of time.

This impressive developmental activity has been described by anthropologists as 'external gestation' or 'the fourth stage'. In order to complete this successfully, Nature requires the immature human infant to be kept close to and protected by the mother until the body systems have sufficiently developed. The equivalent in the marsupial world is the baby kangaroo, or joey, kept in its mother's pouch until it is ready to manage the world on its own.

The obstetric dilemma

So the two crucial developments in our anatomical history that set us apart from other primates are our larger brains and the ability to walk upright. But are these things at odds with each other when it comes to childbirth? This is the so-called 'obstetric dilemma': large brains and the larger skulls that encase them need a roomier pelvis to pass through at birth, but the resulting wider pelvis may then not adapt well to bipedal walking.

There is a belief that women's ability to give birth has been compromised because of these developments and that the two elements conflict with each other. Part of Nature's compromise has been to reduce the length of pregnancy in humans to get around this 'design fault', but this means that babies are, in effect, born 'too early', in order to ensure they don't get stuck.

On the other hand, there are plenty of people who don't accept that hypothesis and believe that the idea that there's an inbuilt difficulty experienced during human birth is a myth.[51] They argue that the evolution of encephalisation, combined with a narrower, re-orientated birth canal, may have led to the potential for complications in the birthing process but that these changes in themselves have not made birth overall any more 'difficult' for Homo sapiens. If anything, they are unique and extremely clever evolutionary adaptations that have enabled women to continue to give birth successfully, despite the 'obstetric challenge'. The evidence for this point of view is the rate at which the human population has expanded.

An interesting piece of research by an anthropologist called Holly Dunsworth was published in 2012 to bolster this argument.[52] She revisited 'the obstetric dilemma' and began searching for the hard evidence to prove the hypothesis, but found this was hard to come by. Yes, these two changes both happened around the same time, but was there a causal link? This is an important question to ask and I will return to it again when I look at the evidence around safety in birth.

In this research, Dunsworth looked at the dilemma in two parts: First, do wider hips prove to be a detriment to walking? She collaborated with fellow anthropologist Anna Warrener, to answer this question. They placed men and women on treadmills at a walking pace, and found that women were just as efficient with their wider hips as the men. They therefore concluded that there was no correlation between wide hips and a diminished ability or 'locomotor economy'. The second element revisited the argument that pregnancy in humans has to be shorter than that in other primates because the larger human skull can no longer fit through the pelvis easily. In fact, Dunsworth found evidence to the contrary: human gestation is not actually shorter, if anything, it is slightly longer than in other primates, and human babies are, in fact, slightly bigger than has been hypothesized, not smaller.

What Dunsworth and Warrener discovered is that for mammals in general – and this includes humans – the length and weight of the baby tended to be predicted by the mother's body size. Because body size is a good proxy for an animal's metabolic rate and function, Dunsworth wondered if metabolism might offer a better explanation for the timing of human birth than the pelvis shape and size.

They then teamed up with other researchers and scientists to look at human physiology and 'energetics', and came up with a new hypothesis for the timing of birth. They called it the 'EGG' hypothesis – 'Energetics, Gestation, Growth'.

In this hypothesis, babies are born when they're born because there is a limit to the number of calories a woman can burn in any day, and during pregnancy she slowly heads towards that energetic ceiling until she reaches the limit of her maximum energy output for her baby's continued growth. Once she reaches that point, it will precipitate her going into labour. Her energy, therefore, is the primary evolutionary constraint to continued pregnancy, not the width of her hips. When you look at the metabolic data on offer, research suggests that women give birth when they are about to cross into a metabolic 'danger zone'.

If this theory is true, it could also provide a further explanation as to why human babies are so helpless compared to primates. A chimpanzee baby is able to crawl at around one month old, for example, whereas a human baby doesn't crawl until around seven months. If we were to give birth to a newborn baby that was at the same developmental level as a chimpanzee, it would require a 16-month gestation. This would take mothers well past their 'energetic' limit and into the metabolic danger zone.

Dunsworth's conclusion is that we have been fed a rather warped anthropological view of women's development, namely that the male pelvis is the ideal form, while the female pelvis is less than ideal because of childbirth. And yet she argues:

> The female births the babies. So if there's an ideal, it's female, and it's no more compromised than anything else out there. Selection maintains its adequacy for locomotion and for childbirth. If it didn't, we'd have gone extinct.
>
> ScienceDaily (2012)[53]

The reason I'm including this debate here is because I believe the obstetric dilemma is indicative of a sort of universal anxiety about our ability to 'do' birth that has come to dominate thinking around safety and place of birth. Over time, and through the increasingly restrictive prism of 'risk management', the idea that somehow the baby won't fit became another reason for women to deliver in hospital, just in case. Although it has since become much less common, when I was a student midwife 20 years ago, the recommendation of a caesarean section because of worries that the baby might be too big, and therefore would be unable to fit through the pelvis, was quite commonplace. Known as cephalopelvic disproportion (CPD), this approach undoubtedly contributed to the alarming increase in caesarean section rates through the 1970s, with many of them proving unnecessary as very normal-sized babies were then delivered by surgery.

Another pendulum swing in more recent years means that nowadays the test for suspected CPD is to labour anyway and, if the baby is genuinely too big to fit through his or her mother's pelvis, her labour simply won't progress. Equally, there can be some surprisingly successful combinations ... I was well over 5kg (11lb) in weight when I arrived safely and without drama in my mother's bedroom three days after Christmas 1954. She was all of 1.57m (5 feet 2 inches), with size 3 feet, but clearly had no problem pushing me out.

So, if we accept Holly Dunsworth's hypothesis, perhaps we can revisit and reframe the misguided perception that women are poorly designed to give birth and argue instead that we are, for the most part, perfectly well shaped and capable of giving birth to our babies, but we need optimal conditions in which to do so – and that perhaps it is the lack of those that cause so many of the problems women appear to experience in the modern childbirth of the 20th century.

Normal birth and changing lifestyles

If we can surmise that, since our adaptation to bipedalism, the physiological process of labour and birth hasn't changed that much, we certainly can't say the same for women's lifestyles – at least, not in the 'developed' nations. Early prehistoric hunter-gatherer communities were tightly bound together and lived close to Nature, in harmony with its rhythms and the changing seasons. Life was brutal and harsh in many ways, and the weakest members were simply unable to reproduce or survive, minimising the number of flawed or damaged genes that could be passed on. In general, women were physically far fitter and healthier than they are today, accustomed as they were to daily physical labour and surviving on a diet free from any processed foods, refined sugar or chemicals.

For this reason, childbirth was probably easier for our ancient ancestors, who would recover quickly because they had support from the community (it was a group responsibility to care for newborns). The prehistoric view of birth was more woman-centred than child-oriented. The birthing woman would be a known and contributive member of her community, embodying knowledge relevant to its day-to-day survival. During labour her physiological, emotional and environmental needs would be recognised and largely met with the support and assistance of other women in her community, and then she in turn would pass on this knowledge and support to the next labouring woman.

Positions in labour

With the onset of bipedalism, the positions in which women gave birth started to adapt to their new, upright stature. Ancient anthropological literature from throughout the world demonstrates that in general, unlike primate mothers, the prevalent way for women to give birth was by vertical delivery.[54] A woman would instinctively choose to be upright and active in her labour, because it is the optimal position for maximising the effect of her expulsive efforts, working with gravity to deliver her baby. What our ancestors did through instinct we have had to research and gather evidence for, but the answer is the same: we can now 'prove' that upright positions such as kneeling, squatting or standing result in a shorter second stage of labour and contribute to the increased likelihood of a more straightforward birth.[55]

In Ancient Egypt, women would usually sit on a primitive birthchair made of bricks, or they would kneel. In the Middle Ages, it was commonplace for women to give birth on a low birthchair while assistants stood on either side or behind to offer support. There were different versions of these birthchairs, depending on the wealth of the woman's family: they could be ornately decorated chairs or simple wooden ones owned by the community and lent out. Anthropological images from Native American Sioux communities depict the woman supported by her partner, standing as she delivers, while her midwife sits behind to catch the child. In some areas of Central Africa, the woman would stand to deliver her baby, supported on either side, while the midwife knelt in front to catch the infant; alternatively, the woman would sit with a midwife applying pressure to her abdomen or pelvis from behind. Meanwhile, members

**Illustration from German doctor Eucharis
Rosslin's 1513 book *Der Rosengarten***

Rosegarten
Das vierd Capitel sagt wie
sich ein yede fraw/in/vo:/vnd nach der geburt halte soll
vnd wie man ir in harter geburt zů hilff kommen soll.

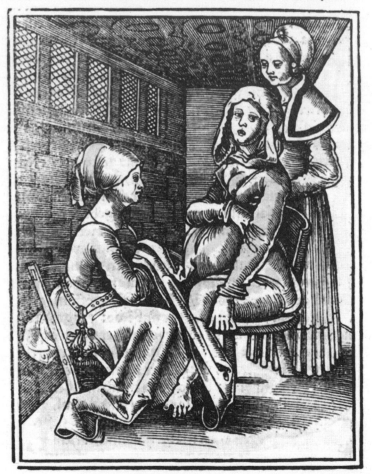

from the community played music nearby for the duration of the labour in order to ward off evil spirits.

Industrialisation and the growth of science in medicine

In the 17th and 18th centuries the cultural and social mores surrounding birth began to undergo a major shift. This occurred first and foremost in the Western world, which had begun to flourish economically with the introduction of industrialisation. The social and political importance of the burgeoning medical and scientific communities grew exponentially and this began to impact on childbirth and the way in which it was 'managed'.

Birth up to this point had always been seen as 'women's work'. Women held the intuitive knowledge to support their sisters and they would then pass this on to the other women who were close to them. Now, though, birth began to be subsumed into the male dominated world of obstetrics, most notably with the publication in 1668 of *Treatise on the Diseases Affecting Women During and Post Partum* by the French obstetrician François Mauriceau.[56]

For the first time, female anatomy and physiology were described in detail, and Mauriceau began to seek solutions for complications in labour in order to reduce the rising mortality rates for mothers and infants. At the end of the 17th century he introduced the obstetric bed, and with it birth became horizontal for the first time – although only for those women with complications because the interventions used to manage them could be done far more easily when a woman was lying down. This development was coupled with the invention of the fetal stethoscope in

1850 to listen to fetal heart tones – these could be heard more clearly and easily when a woman kept still and was on her back. As the frequency in monitoring the fetal heartbeat increased, out of convenience this resulted in more and more women within a hospital environment lying on hospital beds to give birth, even with a normal labour. Over the next century, this shift in practice would prove to have a lasting effect on the birth process in industrialised, developed nations and laid the foundations for what we now call the 'medical model of birth'.

The introduction of hospital-based birth

Hospitals in the 18th and 19th century were generally charitable, 'lying-in' hospitals, used mainly by poorer women who may have had nowhere else to go, or by women having their babies in secret. They were unpopular and viewed as dangerous places in which to give birth due to the high rate of infection and unclean conditions, with many women dying, especially of puerperal infection (a postpartum bacterial infection of the reproductive tract). Since medical attendants did not understand the importance of hand washing, the spread of bacteria was rife in these early institutions.

All other women were still giving birth at home, and in 1900 the home birth rate was 98 per cent. From this point onwards though, this percentage steadily declined until today, over 100 years later, our home birth rate is only 2.3 per cent – almost the exact opposite. If there is now a move to increase the option of home birth for more women again, it is important to understand the reasons why this complete shift in practice occurred in the first place.

From home to hospital timeline

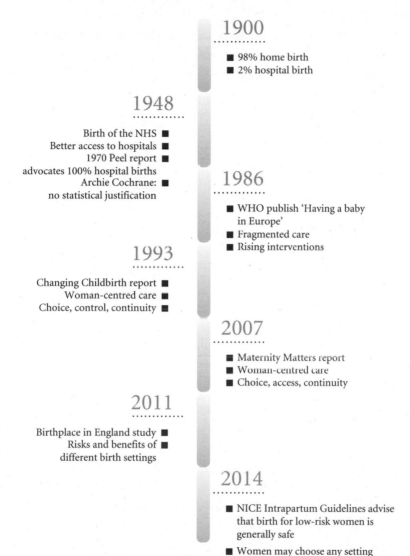

1900

- 98% home birth
- 2% hospital birth

1948

- Birth of the NHS
- Better access to hospitals
- 1970 Peel report advocates 100% hospital births
- Archie Cochrane: no statistical justification

1986

- WHO publish 'Having a baby in Europe'
- Fragmented care
- Rising interventions

1993

- Changing Childbirth report
- Woman-centred care
- Choice, control, continuity

2007

- Maternity Matters report
- Woman-centred care
- Choice, access, continuity

2011

- Birthplace in England study
- Risks and benefits of different birth settings

2014

- NICE Intrapartum Guidelines advise that birth for low-risk women is generally safe
- Women may choose any setting

Birth and its place in modern society

There has been a profound shift in the culture and social context of birth over the last few decades in particular. If there is now a growing awareness that perhaps it is time for the pendulum to swing back, it is important to try to understand the reasons why it went as far as it did, given that our ancestors and more recent forebears were managing to birth their babies perfectly well within their safe and known surroundings and without the accoutrements of modern medicine.

The early signs were there with the increasing obstetric interest in solving the occasional complications of birth, but to be in a position where the vast majority of women now give birth in hospital highlights the remarkable shift in how birth is viewed and managed. These views generally stem from ideas surrounding safety and risk – it was always assumed by most commentators, especially within the medical community, that mortality rates in this country began to decline during the middle decades of the 20th century because that is when women started having their babies in hospital.

A cursory skim through the official data might even appear to back up this presumption, but on closer inspection, this is another case of assuming a causal link between two simultaneous events, which in fact does not exist. It took an extraordinary woman, a statistician called Marjorie Tew, first to realise this and then to try to bring it to everyone's attention with the publication of her book *Safer Childbirth? A Critical History of Maternity Care* (1995).[57] Her conclusions, however, fell largely on determinedly 'deaf ears'. We will revisit and explore them further in the next section.

In the meantime ... back to the early 1900s. Health was becoming a legitimate cause for public concern and, in 1919, the government created the Ministry of Health, complete with a separate department for maternity and child welfare. After the acknowledgment of the appalling conditions of many 'lying-in' hospitals sparked an official enquiry into the high rate of maternal deaths, improvements were made, along with formalising the standards of professional midwives and obstetricians.

Educational and social measures were introduced to improve women's health throughout pregnancy and birth, and Local Authorities began to provide antenatal support to women, as well as creating more maternity homes and steadily increasing the numbers of hospital beds around the country.

In 1927 the first statistics about live births were collected and it was recorded that 15 per cent took place in charitable hospitals and maternity homes. Ten years later, in 1937, this figure had more than doubled to 35 per cent.

The Second World War was partly responsible for the increase in hospital births in the 1940s. More women wanted to have their babies in hospital – out of convenience as much as a concern for safety. At a time when resources were extremely scarce, it would have been a luxury to be given a bed and to be able to access food provisions that weren't coming out of your own very limited rations. And so, by 1946, 54 per cent of all births were taking place in hospital.

After the Second World War, the creation of the NHS in 1948 ensured that free medical care was available to all users at their time of need. Funded by collected general and local taxes along with compulsory health insurance, the NHS was built on the premise that health was now a national responsibility. Better-access hospitals were created and the government of the day began to introduce new health policies and regulations.

One of these new regulations meant that the first point of contact for a pregnant woman was a GP rather than a midwife, a decision that was to have a lasting impact on the level of control midwives had in determining maternity care policies. Steadily, the midwife's lead role in birth appeared to be dwindling, and midwives were increasingly assisting doctors with the birth, or 'delivery' rather than conducting it themselves, i.e. more in the role of an obstetric nurse than a midwife. As the midwife's status fell, so did the number of home births she attended.

Following the creation of the NHS, the new policies being written for maternity were principally concerned with and focused on where the birth should take place, with hospitals being increasingly cited as the preferred option. This in turn led to a steady growth in the number of hospital deliveries and with it the wider application and acceptance of an increasingly medicalised approach to birth over the next few decades.

In 1956 the Guillebaud Inquiry into the financial cost of the NHS identified a 'state of confusion'[58] within the maternity services, and an early review was recommended. This resulted in the publication of the Cranbrook Committee Report in 1959. Medical opinion suggested that more women should be classified as 'high risk' due to new obstetric knowledge and methods, and in many hospitals the supply of hospital beds did not match the demand. In the light of this proposal, the Cranbrook Report recommended a target of 'sufficient hospital beds to provide for a national average of 70 per cent of all births to take place in hospital ... this should be adequate to meet the needs of all women in whose case histories the balance of advantage appears to favour confinement in hospital'.[59]

Because there were low-risk as well as high-risk pregnant women being included in this 70 per cent, as a consequence their births came to be viewed and managed in much the same way. The Cranbrook Report also included recommendations that continued to diminish the midwife's authority in the birth setting, stating that 'a general practitioner obstetrician should, whenever possible, attend all domiciliary confinements, to safeguard the mother and baby against unforeseen emergencies'.[60] The primary skills of the midwife were being sidelined as 'domiciliary' in favour of the more respected clinical role of the consultant obstetrician or doctor.

Despite an increase in the birth rate over the same period, this average of 70 per cent hospital births was achieved by 1965, and by 1968 it had risen to 79 per cent. The increase in numbers of hospital births was possible because of a simultaneous reduction in the length of time a woman would normally stay in hospital postnatally, which by this point was an average of 6.6 days – dropping from the previous standard of 10 days. The Cranbrook Report had actually rejected this option and wanted it to remain as 10 days for all women, but in the end it was a question of necessity.

As the trend towards a hospital birth setting increased, so did the numbers of hospital midwives, while the need for community midwives declined. The number of smaller, stand-alone maternity homes based in the community also declined as policy preference was for an increase in the number of larger hospitals with large consultant units, taking women from a wider area.

The increasing medicalisation of birth

When I use the term 'medicalisation', I am referring to the process in which human conditions, such as childbirth, come to be redefined as medical conditions. Medical conditions are generally seen as requiring treatment, and so a second phenomenon, 'pharmaceuticalisation', follows closely behind, in which drugs are researched, developed and marketed to treat the medical condition. This is true not only of childbirth of course, as there are now any number of 'medicalised' human conditions on offer – for example, obesity and grief-related depression are two examples that are now both treatable through medication and surgery.

But there is something unique about the process of growing and birthing a baby, which over time has come to play a particularly powerful role in the cultural rite of passage for young women, and which, as a midwife, I believe has a strong element of, and potential for, empowerment and self-development. Labour is not easy. It can be very challenging, and you usually need to draw on your inner resources to get through it. But when successfully negotiated, labour can also provide a rich vein of personal resources on which to draw over the following years, not least through the many and varied challenges of parenting.

Looking back over the years with the benefit of hindsight, we can trace enormous changes, beginning with many new obstetric practices from 1965, which led to further, overwhelming changes in maternity care. These have all had profound and probably largely unintended consequences on women's attitudes and approaches to childbirth.

The most significant of these changes were mainly instigated by the Report of the Peel Committee in 1970, led by consultant obstetrician John Peel. The Peel Report advocated for all births to take place in a medical setting, recommending that 'sufficient facilities should be provided to allow for 100 per cent hospital delivery'. Going even further, it stated that 'the greater safety of hospital confinement for mother and child justifies this objective'.[61]

What now seems extraordinary is that during this entire period there was no statistical evidence in each new report to support the recommendation that it was safer for all women to give birth in hospital. Indeed, the Peel Report was challenged over the basis of its far-reaching conclusions and was heavily criticised for its lack of evidence. It also came under fire for failing to listen to or reflect the voices and experiences of the women who used the service. Yet despite this, the Peel Report was a powerful player in the politics and policies of the time and it contributed enormously to the dramatic shift over the next decade from home to hospital.

Between 1963 and 1972 the proportion of hospital deliveries increased from 68 per cent to 91 per cent; and from 1975 to the late 1990s it didn't fall below 95 per cent. Since then there has been a slow but steady rise of midwife-led birth centres. Although these are mostly 'alongside'(i.e. within the hospital grounds and sometimes right next door to) the obstetric unit, the more holistic philosophy and focus on an unmedicalised birth, which such places have to varying degrees, is beginning to make a difference to outcomes.

Back to the 1970s, though, and the status of the midwife waned even further as the delivery and management of maternity care was advocated by obstetric teams (the Peel Report recommended that 'small isolated obstetric units should be replaced by larger, combined consultant and general practitioner units in general hospitals'). The number of consultants present at births steadily rose as the rate of interventions over this period increased dramatically.

The role of medicalisation in birth in the United Kingdom was now firmly established, with maternity care in hospitals increasingly fragmented and interventions a routine feature of labour and birth. Caesarean sections, oxytocic drugs to induce labour and episiotomies (a surgical incision to enlarge the vaginal opening) became commonplace in many consultant units. Antenatal care was also transformed, with the introduction of ultrasound scanning, initially used to diagnose and confirm high-risk births, gradually becoming a standard in all pregnancies. Ultrasound, just like so many of the practices brought in over these years, has never been subjected to rigorous research as to its benefits or side effects and is now far too universally accepted to roll back, even if we wanted to.[62]

Safety and place of birth

By the 1980s the narrative and debate in maternity care was largely focused around safety, and in 1982 the government set up the Maternity Services Advisory Committee to the Secretary of State for Social Services, whose report stated that 'the practice of delivering nearly all babies in hospital has contributed to the dramatic reduction in stillbirths and neonatal deaths'[63] The report concluded that all births carried medical risks, so it strongly reinforced the recommendation from the Peel Report – that hospital was the safest place to be. It was during the 1980s that the rate of home birth dropped to what would be its lowest point – below 1 per cent.

This was probably the point at which the state of counter-productivity was reached, defined as when the institutions of advanced industrial society reach a certain threshold and cease to be useful and their activities begin to go against their stated aims. As medicalisation peaked and the conditions in which it was administered began to take their toll on the resilience of women and their caregivers, the result was an increase in a number of outcomes that were far from helpful for many people. In fact, this had been the case for a long time, as the work of Tew demonstrates.[64] But realisation only dawned in the late 20th century that the 'system' administering our maternity service did not work and that although mortality rates were comparatively low, this was not the whole story (i.e. the reasons behind this state of affairs were not necessarily the ones everyone had assumed). The counter argument, that childbirth – along with the other human 'conditions' of death and mental illness – did not belong in a system of 'industrialised' institutional care, began to resonate with more and more people.

The ongoing and often fierce debate surrounding the provision of maternity care was ignited during this time and quickly became extremely polarised, as it still is today, between those who argue for minimal intervention in a supportive, home environment (or a birth centre) away from the clinical hospital setting, and those who believe modern birth technologies are necessary and that a hospital setting is essential for a safe delivery. Women unwillingly and unwittingly became stereotyped if they voiced a desire to choose a certain type of birth – whether that was a natural birth or a planned caesarean.

Opposition to the 'institutionalising' of childbirth had always existed, with natural birth advocates (notably, the late Sheila Kitzinger) and nascent maternity pressure groups arguing that the over-medicalisation of the normal process of birth was not a universally positive experience for women – indeed far from it – and that women should take back 'control' of their births and not be routinely subjected to humiliating procedures such as shaving and enemas. Their campaign became increasingly vocal as dissatisfaction levels grew and the importance and influence of a more evidence-based approach to the debate began to gain ground.

The National Childbirth Trust (NCT), which was initially set up in 1958 as the Natural Childbirth Trust and changed its name in 1961, taught classes and ran workshops to prepare women and their partners for childbirth. It promoted a reduction in routine interventions and argued for a more homely environment within hospital labour wards, and tried to work, albeit largely unsuccessfully at first, with the medical establishment to provide for more home births for low-risk women. The Association for Improvements in Maternity Services (AIMS) was also established in 1960, with a mission to fight for a woman's right to autonomy and choice and for women to receive kinder, more dignified and respectful care from the establishment. These organisations are still thriving today and continue to campaign for and facilitate improved care and better choices for women within the maternity services.

The sustained criticism of maternity care eventually led to government policy changes in the 1990s that now began to focus much more on the needs of women. In 1993 the Expert Maternity Group was set up to examine and address the issues and to recommend any changes that were needed. The result was the report, *Changing Childbirth*, published by the Department of Health in the same year, which heralded a significant shift in thinking by promoting women-centred care in maternity services through an increase in the three 'Cs': choice, continuity and control.[65]

The findings and conclusions of *Changing Childbirth* were in direct opposition to the Peel Report, which had imagined a future in maternity care with significantly less choice of where and how women could give birth. *Changing Childbirth* highlighted the importance of listening to women and challenged the concept of rigid protocols that resulted in many unwanted and unnecessary interventions in the name of safety.

What is interesting to note, with hindsight, is how effective the Peel Report was in changing behaviour and, in comparison, what little effect the more recent policies and evidence seem to have made in turning the tide of medicalisation. Although there have been some significant changes in process, so that lots of procedures that were simply done without question – or consent – have gone, many of them go hand in hand with societal changes, such as the greater recognition in law of an individual's human rights. There is some evidence though that there is still often great resistance to women choosing their own path, with increased levels of bullying and coercion being reported to some of the organisations mentioned above.

Perhaps the reason why a reversal of the position that high levels of intervention and a hospital setting must be safer is harder to achieve than the other way around is because of the loss of confidence surrounding birth, both for women and midwives. With the introduction of medicalisation in birth, the seeds of fear around childbirth were also planted. The continued assertion through the 1970s and 1980s that birth had various medical risks attached to it and that the process of giving birth itself was inherently dangerous has inevitably caused a concomitant rise in anxiety and fear attached to both the level of pain involved and the risk of death or injury to either mother or baby. Alongside the loss of confidence about women's ability to safely and straightforwardly give birth to their babies without any 'help', there has been a slow and steady rise in litigation. As the risk of being sued has increased, with all the stress and fear that that process engenders, the response has been an increase in intervention – 'just in case' – because it is safer to be seen as 'doing something' than be accused of failing to take action to prevent a tragedy.

This element of fear inevitably dominated the debate when it came to choosing where to give birth, and clear, informed and unbiased information on choice often didn't trickle down to local policy, or at the first point of contact a woman had with the NHS. This was despite a joint statement released by the Royal Colleges representing obstetricians, midwives and general practitioners in 1992:

> Clear and unbiased information about the options for ante-natal care and the place of delivery should be provided wherever a woman makes first contact with the health service.

The woman's own views and references should be a very significant factor in formulating any programmes of care. It has to be recognized that these may not always coincide with the opinions of her professional adviser.

As cited in Tew (1998)[66]

The intentions of this statement couldn't be clearer, but still it hasn't translated into practical action and solutions even 23 years on. In 2007 the Department of Health published another document entitled *Maternity Matters*, which again called for further choice to be offered to women in the type of care and place of birth, but these policies have yet to be fully implemented.[67]

An NCT report conducted in 2011 found that almost 20 years on from *Changing Childbirth*, women are still very restricted in their choices, with only a minority of births taking place in midwife-led units or at home.[68] This is in spite of these environments being known to be safe for low-risk women, with much better outcomes and certainly more cost-effective than births taking place in large, consultant-led units.

My own journey into midwifery came during a time of increasing awareness that a shift in culture and attitude was needed with regard to how we manage birth in the United Kingdom. I started training in 1995, and the excitement and sense of change that the *Changing Childbirth* report had created was palpable. There were a number of continuity-of-care pilot schemes, following on from Caroline Flint's successful '*Know your Midwife*' randomised control study in south-west London in the mid-1980s,[69] and in 1994 the South-East London Midwifery Group Practice, which later changed its name to

'Albany', was set up. This was an innovative new scheme linked to a GP surgery, and was set up by an independent group practice of midwives who negotiated a contract with King's College Hospital to provide continuity of care for women in the community. As I qualified in 1998 and started work at King's College Hospital in London, it seemed to me that there was a new way of working being introduced, a relationship-focused model of care, based much more on a partnership with the women and their families. Sadly though, and for a myriad of reasons, this vision of a brave new world for maternity services did not put down sufficiently robust roots to take hold. Instead, over the intervening years, what I (and many others) consider to be a risk-averse, bureaucratic and hierarchical model of care – with the majority of births taking place in obstetric units – has, if anything, increased its dominance.

I resigned from my post in the NHS six months after starting and took the decision to go into independent practice with a determination to campaign for more women-centred, continuity of carer models within the NHS. I'm still doing that 17 years later but with a renewed sense of hope that perhaps the changes that are coming this time around will be more sustainable because we've learnt the lessons from before.

Stats, facts and false conclusions

I have already mentioned Marjorie Tew. I now want to explain and discuss her work further because, for me, what she did was illustrate clearly, logically and irrefutably, just how easy it is to take two sets of statistical 'facts' about separate events that happen to occur at the same time and make the fundamental mistake of assuming a causal link where, in fact, none exists. Her seminal work, *Safer Childbirth? A Critical History of Maternity Care* (first published in 1990, with a second edition in 1998),[70] should, in my humble opinion, be required reading by every healthcare professional working in maternity services as well as by every policy-maker and parent-to-be. If you are interested, it is well worth acquiring your own copy for an engrossing and educational read.

By way of background, in 1975 Tew was a research statistician and was working as a tutor at Nottingham University's medical school. She was teaching her students how to use official statistics to find out about various conditions and found herself genuinely confused by some of the results. Much to her surprise, she discovered that none of the official data supported the widely held view that increased hospitalisation was the reason for the decline in the maternal and infant mortality rates over the same period. Intrigued, she did further research, which confirmed that, far from being the cause of the reduced rates of maternal and infant mortality, the increased hospitalisation of mothers in labour and the greater use of interventions that went hand in hand with that, was in fact linked to *more* morbidity in low-risk mothers and their babies – not less. As Sheila Kitzinger wrote in the Foreword of the second edition of Tew's *Safer Childbirth?*:

Home is as safe as hospital for women who are at low risk. Moreover, if low risk women give birth in hospital they are more likely to have complicated births and be ill afterwards.

Tew (1998)[71]

Having combed the global research thoroughly, Tew could find no evidence to support the idea that medical interventions made birth safer for most mothers and their babies and found that, in fact, many cause harm. The conclusion she arrived at, having thoroughly analysed all the available facts and figures, was that childbirth is best managed without direct human intervention and that the key to successful birth is first and foremost the good health of the parents, especially the mother. Nutrition, poor living environments, poverty and neglect etc. are the real enemies, and when they are tackled, together with improved basic hygiene and limiting the spread of disease, then overall health improves and mortality rates start to fall.

And this is exactly what happened in the United Kingdom. Mortality rates here were starting to fall *over the same time period* as more women were being admitted into hospital to have their babies. The key to this was not that women were now in a safer place and having increasing amounts of interventions but that there were better living conditions and improvements in public health policy. What Tew does in her book is present the factual evidence to demonstrate this.

Mothers and their babies continue to die in unacceptably high numbers across the developing world due to conditions of extreme poverty combined with cultural traditions such as early marriage. These issues must be tackled if we are to see global maternal mortality rates improve. Of course, good midwifery and obstetric care are also crucial, but in order to really make a difference these interventions need to be provided in combination with improved living conditions, not in isolation.

Tew's theory as to why hospital and interventions don't actually improve outcomes should not come as a surprise to those of us who believe that birth is so much more than just a physical activity. She argues in her book that, without the emotional and social elements being in tune with and driving the physical process via the endocrine or hormonal system, labour will simply not be as efficient or as straightforward. She came to the conclusion that the modern delivery ward makes it almost impossible to create the optimal conditions for birth, especially where an atmosphere of 'danger and fear' is linked to and permeates the space where women are labouring.

With the more recent evidence of the Birthplace study[72] and others adding to the debate, Tew's meticulous research and analysis should finally get the recognition it deserves because the same conclusions have been reached by this new research. And this time they have been included as the basis for the NICE intrapartum guidance published in late 2014.[73]

These national recommendations – that 'out of hospital' birth should be actively promoted among healthy women without complicating factors – will feel counter-intuitive to many people, especially as we have had the concept of safety so strongly linked to hospital birth for many decades. But, if there is consensus that our maternity services should be founded on the best available evidence (and who would disagree with that premise?), we should be basing the provision of that service on what the evidence tells us.

Ensuring that women have much greater access to out of hospital options, whether at home or in birth centres, is going to be key to improving outcomes as well as improving the experience for both healthy women and for those with additional complications, because then the care that both groups receive will be better tailored to their needs.

None of this is new information and, over the years, there have been many initiatives and proposals, including the *Changing Childbirth* report and the Association of Radical Midwives' (ARM) *New Vision* for the future of maternity services (first written in 1986 and then revised in 2013),[74] to try to reverse the relentless increase in intervention rates and to strengthen the role of the midwife as the lead professional in normal birth for healthy women without complications.

To date, though, none of these initiatives has managed to succeed at a national level and indeed, the rates of interventions and caesarean section have continued to climb. The culture of fear surrounding pregnancy and birth has, if anything, intensified, not just for women having babies but, even more worryingly, among many of the midwives and obstetricians who provide their care. The cause of this fear in the caregivers themselves may be based on many different factors: perhaps feeling anxious about having a poor outcome and the possibility of being blamed for it; being concerned about not spotting a problem developing (more likely when you not familiar with a woman's history); worries about being reprimanded for not following guidelines or not knowing about all the obstetric unit's policies. If the midwives and doctors are feeling anxious, the chances are they will be communicating their anxiety to the woman and her partner, thus intensifying their level of fear in an increasingly downward spiral in which confidence in the birth process is lost and the resulting rise in adrenaline begins to interfere with the labour hormones.[75]

Tew argues that it is this obstetric environment, a product of the technocratic approach to birth, that has, with its focus on physical and medical safety, increased the perception that childbirth is a dangerous time for women and their babies. This emphasis on the individual woman's medical risk factors means that the context of her care, whether organisational or environmental, is rarely considered.

This is a big mistake, according to Tricia Anderson, an inspirational midwife and author, who tragically died of a brain tumour in 2007. She argued passionately that risk-assessment processes are flawed because they do not include or acknowledge the risks that are posed by the deficiencies within a busy obstetric unit or a hard-pressed community team of midwives. Factors such as lack of continuity, poor handovers of care, inexperienced staff having to cope alone during busy periods, as well as the effect of bullying, blaming and defensive practice may all contribute to potential harm and are not automatically included as an important part of the equation in risk assessments for an individual woman.[76]

Staff shortage alert!

What we find now on many labour wards are 'dashboards', which monitor a variety of factors that will 'red flag' problems in real time as a way of trying to ameliorate the risks they pose. If at the beginning of the shift there is a shortage of staff (e.g. because of sickness), this is flagged, and one of the immediate solutions is to contact any community-based midwives, who may be on call for home births, and ask them to come in to cover that shift. Sadly, I'm not sure if a lack of midwives on call for home births would merit a red flag on such a system.

If you are thinking about your options, it is important to consider how the place in which you labour and give birth may affect how your labour unfolds. After weighing up all the facts, you may arrive at the conclusion that being in hospital might not be the right place for you. However, if you decide to plan for a home birth, you need to be aware that, as a choice, it may suddenly not exist if the situation above arises in your area the day you go into labour. At the moment, the default position is invariably that the labour ward is staffed at the cost of community and other services.

If the official stats, as demonstrated by Marjorie Tew, don't actually prove that hospital birth is safer – indeed rather the opposite – how is it we didn't embrace our new understanding of data and revert back to community-based care as quickly as we had moved in the opposite direction?

Tew describes in her book her initial disbelief about how her information was received, having assumed rather naively that everyone would be interested in her revelations, be prepared to acknowledge the widespread misinterpretation of the data and want to set the record straight. Instead, she was pretty much shunned by the 'establishment' and mainstream obstetrics, and initially she struggled to get anywhere in publishing her conclusions on official data.

The reasons why it has proved so difficult to promote an alternative reality are complex and to do with traditional power bases, politics, inertia and 'silo thinking' among the different professions and between different organisations. All these elements should be factored in to any risk analysis from an individual woman's point of view, as opposed to the focus being the other way around.

It is my strong belief that women receiving NHS maternity services and the health professionals providing it are caught up in a bureaucratic and complicated system that has become too large and unwieldy to function well for anyone. Looking at it from a risk and safety perspective, it is hard to see how such a conveyor-belt system can identify and correct the external risk factors, which are probably more likely to impact negatively on the progress and outcomes of normal labour than the potential risk that is identified in an individual woman's medical history. The more we begin to identify what the real underlying issues are, the more likely we are to start to be able to do something about them.

Models of Care and Contemporary Home Birth

Different models of care in today's maternity services

What does birth look like today for many women? The modern birth process in the West is consistently managed from a child-centred perspective. The very term 'childbirth' focuses on the eventual outcome – the birth of the baby, rather than the lengthy process preceding it, which instead has the woman as the focus.

In today's technologically enhanced systems within the Western world, it is only in rare circumstances that the health of the woman and child, unless already compromised, are at serious risk in birth. Unfortunately, in many modern hospital deliveries, there is still a gap between the evolved needs of women during labour and delivery and the current conveyor-belt system designed to meet those needs.

Too often, continuity of care is ignored and women still give birth in unfamiliar surroundings with unfamiliar people and are very likely to receive some form of unnecessary intervention. During labour, the delivery of a healthy baby can become the sole objective and focus of everyone's attention, and the role of the woman is too often reduced to passive onlooker, with her emotional and social needs overlooked and often neglected. This happens just at the very time when it is crucial that she receives good personal support – especially since we know that the roots of this assistance are as ancient as our human lineage.

Given our long evolutionary history, with its focus on the emotional wellbeing of the pregnant woman and our intuitive emotional knowledge of childbirth, it is not surprising that many women are frequently left with feelings of disappointment; and an increasing number can be left deeply traumatised by their birth experience within the current modern medical model.

When researching and exploring what we know or can surmise about women's attitudes towards birth over the ages, our female ancestors from prehistoric and ancient cultures did not fear or lack confidence in birth in the way we do now. Childbirth was seen as a totally natural process that was often witnessed by children, and younger women would be told powerful birthing stories by other women in their communities, which led to a greater understanding of the birth process. A woman in labour would be firmly at the centre of her experience and in control of her birth.[77]

The process would be led by her instinctual knowledge, along with her actions, assertiveness and total acceptance of what was happening to her body, while those assisting and supporting her would facilitate this. The authoritative and intuitive knowledge passed on from woman to woman throughout the generations has been transferred elsewhere, and there is now an inherent, normalised belief that childbirth is something to be feared and women need assistance to give birth. Medical intervention is now accepted as the norm because the perception is that there are just too many risks associated with birth and why should or would women endure the pain of labour if there are ways of relieving it with drugs?

This perception, however, is being challenged by a renewed understanding, backed by further research and evidence, that more than just physical care is necessary to ensure a 'safe' birth in its full, holistic sense. My firm belief is that birth as a process needs to be viewed once more as physiological, psychological and primitive in its nature, and that on her journey through pregnancy, birth and beyond, a woman should be accompanied all the way by her 'support team' – midwives who can respond intuitively and compassionately to her many and varied needs and can help her prepare for becoming a mother.

The biomedical model of care

The term 'biomedical' refers to a model of care in which the biology, physiology or anatomy elements connected to birth are paramount and are closely linked to the knowledge generated by medical science. Understanding and supporting the physical aspect of birth is crucial, of course, but it is not the only story. The fundamental problem with this model is that it has largely ignored the other vital but less tangible aspects: the social, emotional or psychological elements of birth. These are much more interwoven into a social model of care, which we will return to later.

Over the past 50 years or so, as the biomedical or techno-cratic model of maternity care has expanded, it has massively increased a process-driven approach to pregnancy and birth in which progress is measured against a set of expectations and then steps are taken to start labour off, speed it up or intervene when the pregnancy or labour doesn't meet those predeter-mined expectations. In order to decide what these parameters are, though, someone has to quantify what is normal: when *should* labour start? How long should it last? Can we differenti-ate between what is pathological delay in one woman's labour and completely normal progress in another without intervening in both situations 'just in case'?

The biomedical approach has to assume that childbirth is a potentially pathological process, with the birth only confirmed as 'normal' in retrospect. The starting position is that there are many risks involved of things 'going wrong' both during the development of the fetus and the baby's passage out into the world. It follows that these risks can be mitigated by a range of different screening tests, monitoring and then, if necessary, an intervention of some sort when there is a deviation from the 'norm', however that is defined.

Although the logic behind such a system is understandable, the reality of trying to measure each woman against a universal 'norm' divided into different risk categories is that it does not take into account the multitude of individual variations that start to become apparent when you try to apply it to real women in the real world. When caring for a pregnant woman, it is crucial that every healthcare provider in the system uses their clinical judgement to adapt and process the information they are being given to take into account the particular circumstances of each woman. This is what 'individualised care' means and, when done well, it can bring together the best of all worlds. Discussing what impact a physical condition may have on a woman's pregnancy is important but it is only the first step. Understanding what else is going on in her life, the level of stress she may be under and what her resilience and coping mechanisms are will be just as important when planning her care and supporting her to make the choices and decisions that will be the most appropriate and safest for her.

A good example of this is a woman who has had a previous caesarean section following a catalogue of interventions in her first pregnancy and who is really wanting to do things differently second time around. The guidelines for vaginal birth after caesarean (VBAC) recommend continuous monitoring with CTG, having a cannula in the back of your hand 'just in case' and strict parameters on how long it is safe for you to labour for. If this woman has already experienced these interventions first time around, she may be anxious about how they will affect her again. She may feel under pressure to 'perform' within the imposed time limit and knows that the monitor will restrict her movements. These are not then the conditions most conducive to enabling her to relax into her labour and work with it in as productive and effective way as possible. When she has an empathetic midwife or doctor who understands the importance of doing things differently this time around, it is then perfectly possible to agree together a plan of care that recognises the risks but also takes into account her previous experience and her preferences for this labour. It may be that she would like to labour in water and would prefer the baby to be monitored with a less intrusive handheld monitor or Sonicaid®. Given that the evidence on the effectiveness of continuous monitoring has yet to be proved, combined with the effect of feeling empowered and enabled in her choices, the chances are that her labour and birth will be safe and have a good outcome – a normal birth and a very positive experience for the mother. There are many other benefits that flow on from this – bonding, breastfeeding, reduced risk of postnatal depression, to name but a few.

The difficulty with the current system of maternity care is that it is essentially a reductionist approach in which, especially when under pressure of time and resources, healthcare professionals often use the processes (guidelines, protocols and policies) without introducing *individual* clinical judgement. In other words, there is a tendency to apply the 'rules' in an uncritical way, without taking into account, and sometimes without even asking, the opinion of the woman in front of them.

Coupled with this over-reliance on protocols and policies is the increased use of litigation, which has become a hugely expensive element of maternity costs within the NHS. The anxiety about being sued has only increased the tendency to try to control every part of the process – there is a belief nowadays that if an adverse outcome occurs, someone must be to blame, which is neither automatically true nor a helpful stance to take. It encourages the belief that, if you are seen to be doing something, then you cannot be accused of having done nothing, and so increases the intervention rate, not necessarily for the right reasons or with better outcomes as a result. We have to acknowledge that modern medicine will never be able to remove all risk from the process of growing and birthing a baby. There is a real tension between managing the process as safely and responsively as possible, in equal partnership with women, while accepting that sometimes, with the best care in the world, poor outcomes do happen and no one is to blame.

There is a balance to be struck here though ... *The Report of the Morecombe Bay Investigation* in 2015 highlighted what can go wrong if any one philosophy or mindset takes precedence.[78] It describes in detail the systematic failures of a service that had become totally dysfunctional and in which the parents whose babies had died had to fight to get the answers they needed. Communication between the different professional groups appeared to have failed on every level and there were ongoing and serious conflicts that affected the relationships across the whole multidisciplinary team. These were deeply divisive and had a hugely detrimental impact on the care that was provided.

We need to ask whether the dysfunctional and damning culture that appears to have flourished at Morecombe Bay is more likely to happen within the 'industrialised' system we have put in place. Where there is a conveyor-belt approach to childbirth, with a women processed through the event, with any number of different individuals looking after her and scant regard given to her partner or to the wider social network and situation she is in, the service is more likely to be fragmented and impersonal. A fragmented service is much more open to communication failures because there are so many more opportunities for miscommunication, even where there are the best of intentions. Within a detached and disconnected work-force, the opportunity and temptation to build mini-fiefdoms and to work in 'silos' means that difficulties within the service are much more likely to occur and it is difficult to challenge and penetrate such a culture once it has taken hold.

Following the *Mid Staffordshire Report*[79] in 2013 and now *Morecombe Bay*, the need for a much more open and transparent culture across the whole of the NHS is apparent. It should be normal practice for healthcare professionals to say sorry, for mistakes to be acknowledged and then the lessons learnt to be disseminated across the service. The challenge is how to introduce this practice into the culture of regulation, inspection and public shaming that currently encourages individuals to hide their mistakes and does nothing to reward clinicians who come forward to share their stories.

This focus on risk has also had the perhaps unintended consequence of fuelling our fears and feeding into our natural instincts to want to protect our babies from the unknown. The result is that the majority of babies in the United Kingdom who are designated as 'low risk' are born in obstetric units even though their birth journey should not, in theory, require any of the range of interventions that are on offer in them. It is especially inappropriate now that we know that the outcomes for these women and their babies are, in fact, better when they take place out of hospital – either in birth centres or, for second or subsequent babies, at home.

The social model of maternity care

The social model of maternity care is one rooted in a more holistic and integrated approach to providing that care, in which the emotional, psychological and social elements of pregnancy and childbirth are given equal weight to the physical aspects. From a risk-management perspective, this would mean that assessing your particular 'risk' factors and considering what will keep you and your baby safe is not just limited to and focused on your medical history. It uses a much more detailed and individualised analysis to try to balance the risks and benefits of one course of action over another in your particular circumstances.

Perhaps the timing is now right for implementing this type of care more widely. We are arriving at a very different stage in human societal organisation as we move from an industrial era into a more information-driven economy where knowledge is a much more universally shared concept and not held just in the hands of the 'professionals'. As more information is freely shared and becomes openly available to anyone who goes looking, the concept of 'authoritative' knowledge about birth that is not also accessible to women themselves becomes more outdated. Being able to consider and weigh up for yourself the actual risk any particular condition might pose for you, as opposed to the theoretical risk for a defined group of people that might include you by age, gender or other parameters, is more possible now than it ever has been.

The effect of this transfer of knowledge, and the consequent rebalancing of the relationship between women and healthcare professionals, might be that the intuitive and evolutionary knowledge of how to birth, which used to be readily and easily accessed as required and which women still carry within themselves, may begin to reassert itself as the medical model and the last century of male dominance over the birth process begins to wane in influence.

The end result, when combined with the growing awareness within the related healthcare professions that we have somewhat lost our way, could be a maternity service in which the best of both worlds merge to produce a gentler, more humane and ultimately safer model of care. Before that can happen, we need an increased awareness of the often inappropriate and complex language used by the external sources of authoritative knowledge – the midwives and doctors who provide the care – to communicate with the women who receive that care. We need to recognise that it is women, who are daily experiencing the physical and emotional changes pregnancy brings, who are the real 'experts' in their condition. The maternity service needs to enable and support them, by sharing additional information sensitively and appropriately, to manage the process them-selves. We need to develop more of a partnership, based on trust and mutual respect, rather than the patriarchal 'doctor/midwife–patient' relationship that is such an accepted part of the medicalised model. For too long, women, often without properly informed consent, have been unnecessarily 'rescued' from experiencing birth the way that Nature has designed and evolution has developed it. The social model of care will, one hopes, redress the balance, not by dismissing the crucial impor-tance of effective and necessary medical input and knowledge but by using a holistic approach to ensure any interventions are used more sparingly and only when needed or requested.

One of the other driving factors for this change is that the evidence for the value of this type of care has been slowly mounting and it is likely that a tipping point is being reached. I believe that a fundamental change in the way that the maternity services are provided will become inevitable. I think that that this will happen not through another top-down, imposed change but by means of a grassroots, bottom-up, community-based approach that refocuses on the value of small-scale, localised care – one that through information technology and the virtual world of information sharing can be interconnected and linked to a supportive wider system in a networked way.

In this new culture, the majority of healthy pregnant women will no longer have to travel to the large obstetric units to give birth but will be able to opt instead for either a low-tech birthing centre or, increasingly, their own home. Time will tell, but I fervently hope that in 20 years from now we are not repeating the same arguments a third time around but instead will have finally arrived at a place of mutual and respectful understanding where appropriately risk-assessed, humane care is the norm.

Where to Give Birth

Recent Evidence
and Guidance

The updated National Institute for Clinical Excellence Guidelines (NICE) intrapartum guidelines December 2014 Adapted from *CG 190 Intrapartum Care for healthy women and babies*. Manchester: NICE. Available from www.nice.org.uk/CG190. Reproduced with permission.

Giving birth is a life-changing event. The care that a woman receives during labour has the potential to affect her – both physically and emotionally, in the short and longer term – and the health of her baby. Good communication, support and compassion from staff, and having her wishes respected, can help her feel in control of what is happening and contribute to making birth a positive experience for the woman and her birth companion(s).

This guideline covers the care of healthy women who go into labour at term (37^{+0} to 41^{+6} weeks). About 700,000 women give birth in England and Wales each year, of whom about 40 per cent are having their first baby. Most of these women are healthy and have a straightforward pregnancy. Almost 90 per cent of women will give birth to a single baby after 37 weeks of pregnancy, with the baby presenting head first. About two-thirds of women go into labour spontaneously. Therefore most women giving birth in England and Wales are covered by this guideline.

Since the original guideline was published in 2007, the number of women giving birth in England and Wales each year has risen, the rate of intervention (instrumental births and caesarean section) has increased slightly, and there has been some reconfiguration of services. The decision to update the guideline was made based on developments in the NHS and new evidence becoming available that could affect the recommendations from 2007.

It is important that the woman is given information and advice about all available settings when she is deciding where to have her baby, so that she is able to make a fully informed decision. This includes information about outcomes for the different settings. It is also vital to recognise when transfer of care from midwifery-led care to obstetric-led care is indicated because of increased risk to the woman and/or her baby resulting from complications that have developed during labour.

Uncertainty and inconsistency of care has been identified in a number of areas, such as choosing place of birth, care during the latent first stage of labour, fetal assessment and monitoring during labour (particularly cardiotocography compared with intermittent auscultation [listening to sounds within the body]) and management of the third stage of labour. These and other related topics are addressed in this guideline update.

The guideline is intended to cover the care of healthy women with uncomplicated pregnancies entering labour at low risk of developing intrapartum complications. In addition, recommendations are included that address the care of women who start labour as 'low risk' but who go on to develop complications. These include the care of women with pre-labour rupture of membranes at term, care of the woman and baby when meconium is present, indications for continuous cardiotocography, interpretation of cardiotoco-graph traces, and management of retained placenta and postpartum haemorrhage. Aspects of intrapartum care for women at risk of developing intrapartum complications are covered by a range of guidelines on specific conditions (see section 3.2) and a further guideline is planned on the intra-partum care of women at high risk of complications during pregnancy and the intrapartum period.

Place of birth

- Explain to both multiparous [given birth more than once] and nulliparous [not given birth before] women that they may choose any birth setting (home, freestanding mid-wifery unit, alongside midwifery unit or obstetric unit), and support them in their choice of setting wherever they choose to give birth:
- Advise low-risk multiparous women that planning to give birth at home or in a midwifery-led unit (freestand-ing or alongside) is particularly suitable for them because the rate of interventions is lower and the outcome for the baby is no different compared with an obstetric unit.
- Advise low-risk nulliparous women that planning to give birth in a midwifery-led unit (freestanding or along-side) is particularly suitable for them because the rate of

interventions is lower and the outcome for the baby is no different compared with an obstetric unit. Explain that if they plan birth at home there is a small increase in the risk of an adverse outcome for the baby. [**new 2014**]

- Commissioners and providers should ensure that all four birth settings are available to all women (in the local area or in a neighbouring area). [**new 2014**]
- Providers, senior staff and all healthcare professionals should ensure that in all birth settings there is a culture of respect for each woman as an individual undergoing a significant and emotionally intense life experience, so that the woman is in control, is listened to and is cared for with compassion, and that appropriate informed consent is sought. [**new 2014**]
- Senior staff should demonstrate, through their own words and behaviour, appropriate ways of relating to and talking about women and their birth companion(s), and of talking about birth and the choices to be made when giving birth. [**new 2014**]

Maternity services should

- provide a model of care that supports one-to-one care in labour for all women **and**
- benchmark services and identify overstaffing or under-staffing by using workforce planning models and/or woman-to-midwife ratios. [**new 2014**]

Commissioners and providers should ensure that there are

- robust protocols in place for transfer of care between settings (see also section 1.6)

- clear local pathways for the continued care of women who are transferred from one setting to another, including:
  - when crossing provider boundaries
  - if the nearest obstetric or neonatal unit is closed to admissions or the local midwifery-led unit is full. [new 2014]

NICE (2014)[80]

The Birthplace in England Research Programme

The NICE guidelines are based on a range of evidence (Appendix 1b)[81] and include the Birthplace in England research programme,[82] which was published in 2011 and was based on births in NHS hospitals and Trusts in England between 2008 and 2010. It was conducted in order to fill important gaps in the evidence relating to the availability, safety, organisation and costs of maternity services provided for women in labour in four different birth settings:

1. Hospital obstetric units (OUs)
2. Alongside midwifery units situated next to obstetric units (AMUs)
3. Freestanding midwifery units (FMUs)
4. Home

It addressed a number of questions including: 'Are there differences in outcomes for the mother and baby between the different birth settings?' and 'What are the organisational features of the maternity care system that may affect quality and safety of care in different settings?' The study measured safety for mother and baby in different birth settings and showed the following results:

Giving birth is generally very safe

- For 'low risk' women the incidence of adverse perinatal outcomes (intrapartum stillbirth, early neonatal death, neonatal encephalopathy, meconium aspiration syndrome, and specified birth-related injuries including brachial plexus injury) was low (4.3 events per 1,000 births).

Midwifery units appear to be safe for the baby and offer benefits for the mother

- For planned births in freestanding midwifery units and alongside midwifery units there were no significant differences in adverse perinatal outcomes compared with planned birth in an obstetric unit.
- Women who planned birth in a midwifery unit (AMU or FMU) had significantly fewer interventions, including substantially fewer intrapartum caesarean sections, and more 'normal births' than women who planned birth in an obstetric unit.

For women having a second or subsequent baby, home births and midwifery unit births appear to be safe for the baby and offer benefits for the mother

- For multiparous women, there were no significant differences in adverse perinatal outcomes between planned home births or midwifery unit births and planned births in obstetric units.

- For multiparous women, birth in a non-obstetric unit setting significantly and substantially reduced the odds of having an intrapartum caesarean section, instrumental delivery or episiotomy.

For women having a first baby, a planned home birth increases the risk for the baby

- For nulliparous women, there were 9.3 adverse perinatal outcome events per 1,000 planned home births, compared with 5.3 per 1,000 births for births planned in obstetric units, and this finding was statistically significant.

For women having a first baby, there is a fairly high probability of being transferred to an obstetric unit during labour or immediately after the birth

- For nulliparous women, the peri-partum transfer rate was 45% for planned home births, 36% for planned FMU births and 40% for planned AMU births.

For women having a second or subsequent baby, the transfer rate is around 10%

- For women having a second or subsequent baby, the proportion of women transferred to an obstetric unit during labour or immediately after the birth was 12% for planned home births, 9% for planned FMU births and 13% for planned AMU births.

The research findings answered a number of important questions, including the following:

Is it safe for a woman to have her first baby at home?

The study found that a woman having a first baby at home is more likely to have a 'normal birth', but there is a fairly high probability (45%) of her being transferred to hospital during labour or immediately after birth and there appears to be an increased risk of an adverse outcome for the baby (9.3 adverse perinatal outcomes per 1,000 planned home births compared with 5.3 per 1,000 births for births planned in obstetric units).

Are outcomes worse for women who are transferred?

Women transfer for many reasons during labour, sometimes for 'straightforward' reasons such as wanting an epidural, but sometimes because the midwife has concerns about the mother or baby. Because of this, women who transfer, on average, have more labour complications than women who do not transfer. So, although women who transfer have worse outcomes than those who do not, it seems probable that this is mainly due to the medical reason that led to the transfer.

For women who develop complications at home or in a midwifery unit, it is likely that transfer to an obstetric unit where they can receive additional observation, treatment or medical care, is the best way of ensuring a good outcome.

The Birthplace in England Research Programme (NPEU)[83]

The Birthplace cost-effectiveness analysis

The Birthplace study also considered the cost-effectiveness of providing home births. The results have surprised the many people who had assumed that home birth was more expensive. If 'too expensive' is the reason given to you for why a home birth service is not available, you will now be able to quote the following figures, which compare NHS costs in the different settings:

- Total mean costs per 'low risk' nulliparous woman were: OU £2075.2, AMU £1,983.1, FMU £1,912.5 and home £1,793.7.

- Total mean costs per 'low risk' nulliparous woman without complicating conditions at the start of care in labour were: OU £1,940.4, AMU £1932.5, FMU £1,880.7 and home £1,719.0.

- Total mean costs per 'low risk' multiparous woman were: OU £1,142.4, AMU £991.3, FMU £968.9 and home £780.4.

- Total mean costs per 'low risk' multiparous woman without complicating conditions at the start of care in labour were: OU £1076.9, AMU £978.3, FMU £953.7 and home £765.8.

The Birthplace in England Research
Programme (NIHR 2011)[84]

These figures include all NHS costs associated with the birth itself – for example midwifery care during labour and immediately after the birth, the cost of any medical care and procedures needed in hospital, and the cost of any stay in hospital, midwifery unit, or neonatal unit immediately after the birth either by the mother or the baby. The costs for planned home and midwifery unit births take account of interventions and treatment that a woman may receive if she is transferred into hospital during labour or after the birth.

The costs do not include any longer term costs of care.

The Birthplace study background Q and As provide further information:

Why are obstetric unit births more expensive? Don't home births take up more of a midwife's time?

Women having a baby at home or in a midwifery unit typically receive more one-to-one care from a midwife but, despite this, planned birth in an obstetric unit is more expensive overall. This is because hospital overheads tend to be higher and women who plan birth in an obstetric unit tend to have more interventions, such as caesarean section, which are expensive.

Which birth setting is most cost-effective?

A cost-effectiveness analysis compares the cost and health effects of an intervention in order to decide if an intervention represents value for money. Cost-effectiveness analysis is useful when trying to decide if it is worth paying more money for a better outcome (health effect).

The analysis showed that planned birth at home, in a free-standing midwifery unit or an alongside midwifery unit were all cost-saving relative to planned birth in an obstetric unit but effectiveness, and hence cost-effectiveness, depended both on whether the analysis focused on outcomes for the mother or outcomes for the baby, and on whether the woman was having a first or subsequent baby:

- For maternal outcomes ('adverse maternal outcome avoided' and 'normal birth'), planned birth at home was the most cost-effective option.
- For women having a first baby, planned home birth was the most cost-effective option by standard health-economic criteria, despite the fact that outcomes for the baby were, on average, less good.
- For women having a second or subsequent baby, planned home birth was also the most cost-effective option, reflecting the fact that in this group of women, planned home births are cheaper and outcomes for the baby are broadly similar to those in an obstetric unit.

The Birthplace in England Research
Programme Background Q&A guide (NPEU)[85]

Further findings from the Birthplace study

Since the publication of the Birthplace study, further analyses have been done on the data and these were published in August 2015.

The purpose of this follow-on project was to further explore factors influencing interventions, transfers and other outcomes in different settings and to address questions relating to the organisation and delivery of services.

The research was conducted as a series of five complementary studies, each addressing a set of research questions related to a specific topic. I've highlighted one of the most relevant ones below, but you can read through all the findings in the main report.

Is there evidence to suggest that rates of intervention and maternal outcome in planned home births differ in NHS Trusts with a high/low volume of planned home births?

Multiparous 'low risk' women who planned home birth in a trust where numerically more home births took place were significantly more likely to have a normal birth and multiparous women who planned birth in a trust with a higher proportion of home births tended to have lower instrumental delivery rates and higher rates of 'normal' and 'straightforward' birth.

> The Birthplace in England National Prospective Cohort Study: further analyses to enhance policy and service delivery decision-making for planned place of birth.[86]

Note: This was not the case for nulliparous women, but that may be because of the limited number in the home birth sample.

Relevant conclusions from the NICE Guidelines

Home births: The primary Birthplace findings, together with the findings of this study support a policy of increasing provision of home birth services to support multiparous women who wish to plan birth at home.

OU intervention rates: Time of day variations in intervention in planned OU births suggest that non clinical factors may be leading to an 'excess' use of epidurals and augmentation in women labouring during 'office hours'. Obstetric units need to examine whether their delivery ward practices and procedures, or staffing levels and skill mix, contribute to this and implement strategies to promote 'normal birth' and reduce unnecessary interventions.

Births to older nulliparous women: Our findings add to the evidence of a marked age-related increase in interventions, including augmentation, instrumental delivery and intrapartum caesarean section, in nulliparous women. There is a need for further investigation of factors contributing to higher intervention rates at older ages.

Information for women: Women considering where to plan birth can be provided with more detailed information about the risk of transfer and the risk of obstetric intervention.

National Institute for Health and Care Excellence (NICE), *Intrapartum Care for Healthy Women and Babies*[87]

Resources

There is an ever growing resource online and locally for those interested in finding out more about homebirth. Just start searching and you will be amazed! In the meantime, here is a selection (in no particular order) to start you off.

www.nct.org.uk The network of local home birth groups is expanding, sometimes as part of the NCT – just do some research to find your nearest one.

www.which.co.uk/birth-choice Includes information on home birth services locally.

http://homebirthersandhopefuls.com An online support network.

www.neighbourhoodmidwives.org.uk/pregnancy-portal Lots of FAQs and 'bite-sized' information about all aspects of pregnancy, labour and birth and the postnatal period.

http://birthingbetter.org Birthing Better Online Childbirth Preparation Course is an award-winning digital resource.

www.thehypnobirthingassociation.com There are lots of local hypnobirthing teachers, so research in your area.

http://hypnobirthing.co.uk/what-is-hypnobirthing

www.hypnobirthing.com/about/hypnobirthing-techniques-benefits

www.psychologytoday.com/blog/consciousness-matters/201105/
mindfulness-moms-the-basics

www.bemindful.co.uk Mindfulness website with details of local teachers and online courses.

http://www.whattoexpect.com/pregnancy-and-meditation.aspx

http://www.fitpregnancy.com/exercise/prenatal-workouts/
10-benefits-prenatal-yoga

http://www.netdoctor.co.uk/parenting/pregnancy/a9179/the-benefits-of-yoga-in-pregnancy

www.becomingmother.co.uk Yoga, mindfulness and birth education.

www.thesophrologynetwork.co.uk Sophrology is based on a combination of Oriental traditions (Yoga, Zen and Buddhist meditation), Western techniques (relaxation, hypnosis) and philosophies (phenomenology and psychology).

www.positivebirthmovement.org To find your Local Positive birth group.

http://mamacafeuk.com/2015/07/vbac-risks-realities-and-home birth Support for vaginal birth after caesarean (VBAC) and home birth.

http://doula.org.uk Doulas support women and their families during pregnancy, childbirth and early parenthood. This support is practical and emotional but non-medical in nature.

www.apec.org.uk Action on Pre-eclampsia (APEC) aims to raise public and professional awareness of pre-eclampsia, improve care and ease or prevent physical and emotional suffering caused by this condition.

www.birthrights.org.uk Birthrights is the UK's only organisation dedicated to improving women's experience of pregnancy and childbirth by promoting respect for human rights.

www.aims.org.uk Association for the Improvement of Maternity Services (AIMs) works towards normal birth, provides independent support and information about maternity choices, raises awareness of current research on childbirth and related issues and protects women's human rights in childbirth.

www.uk-sands.org Very occasionally, parents experience an unexpected and devastating outcome. Sands is the stillbirth and neonatal death charity. They operate throughout the UK, supporting anyone affected by the death of a baby, working to improve the care bereaved parents receive and promoting research to reduce the loss of babies' lives.

www.countthekicks.org.uk Count the Kicks is a UK registered charity that aims to empower mums-to-be with knowledge and confidence throughout their pregnancy.

References

1   Tew, Marjorie, *Safer Childbirth? A Critical History of Maternity Care* (Free Association Books, 1990, 1998).

2   World Health Organization, Global Health Observatory data repository, Millennium Development Goals 5, Maternal and Reproductive Health, 'Women: data by country.' Available at http://apps.who.int/gho/data/node.main.REPWOMEN39? lang=en. Accessed on 30 January 2016.

3   Zielinski, R., Ackerson, K. and Kane Low, L., 'Planned home birth: benefits, risks, and opportunities.' *International Journal of Women's Health* 7 (2015): 361–77.

4   Department of Health, *Changing Childbirth: Report of the Expert Maternity Group* (Chairman Lady Julia Cumberledge) (HMSO, 1993).

5   Hope, Jenny, 'First-time mothers who opt for home birth face triple the risk of death or brain damage in child' *Daily Mail* (23 November 2011).

6   Brocklehurst, P. *et al.*, (Birthplace in England Collaborative Group), 'Perinatal and maternal outcomes by planned place of birth for healthy women with low risk pregnancies: The Birthplace in England national prospective cohort study.' *British Medical Journal* 343 (2011).

7   Tew, Marjorie, *Safer Childbirth? A Critical History of Maternity Care* (Free Association Books, 1990, 1998).

8   Department of Health (DoH), *National Service Framework for Children, Young People and Maternity Services* (DoH, 2004).

9   Department of Health (DoH), *Maternity Matters: Choice, Access and Continuity of Care in a Safe Service.* (DoH, 2007).

10 National Perinatal Birthplace Epidemiology (NPEU) Unit, Birthplace in England Research Programme. Available at www.npeu.ox.ac.uk/birthplace. Accessed on 29 January 2016.

11 National Institute for Health and Care Excellence (NICE), 'NICE confirms midwife-led care during labour is safest for women with straightforward pregnancies.' Available at www.nice.org.uk/news/press-and-media/midwife-care-during-labour-safest-women-straightforward-pregnancies. Accessed on 30 January 2016.

12 Tew, Marjorie, *Safer Childbirth? A Critical History of Maternity Care* (Free Association Books, 1990, 1998).

13 National Maternity Review Report, 2016. Available at www.england.nhs.uk/ourwork/futurenhs/mat-review. Accessed on 28 February 2016.

14 *Montgomery* v *Lanarkshire Health Board* [2015] UKSC 11, paragraph 93.

15 Sandall, J., Soltani, H., Gates, S., Shennan A. and Devane, D., 'Midwife-led continuity models versus other models of care for childbearing women.' *Cochrane Database of Systematic Reviews* 8 (2013).

16 Sutton, J. and Scott, P., *Understanding and Teaching Optimal Foetal Positioning* (Birth Concepts, 1996).

17 Ahmad, Aishah, 'The Association Between Fetal Position at the Onset of Labour and Birth Outcomes' (PhD thesis, University of Birmingham, 2011). Available at http://etheses.bham.ac.uk/3723/2/Ahmad12PhD.pdf. Accessed on 2 January 2016.

18 Anderson, Tricia, 'Out of the laboratory: back to the darkened room.' MIDIRS *Midwifery Digest* 12(1) (2002): 65–9.

19 Elharmeel, S. M. A., Chaudhary, Y., Tan, S., Scheermeyer E., Hanafy, A. and van Driel, M. L., 'Surgical repair of spontaneous perineal tears that occur during childbirth versus no intervention.' *Cochrane Database of Systematic Reviews* 8 (2011).

20 Jahdi, F., Shahnazari, M., Kashanian, M., Ashghali, M., Farahani, M. A. and Haghani, H., 'A randomized controlled trial comparing the physiological and directed pushing on the duration of the second stage of labor, the mode of delivery and Apgar score.' *International Journal of Nursing and Midwifery* 3(5) (2011): 55–9.

21 Janssen, P., Farah Shroff, F. and Jaspar, P., 'Massage therapy and labor outcomes: A randomized controlled trial.' *International Journal of Therapeutic Massage and Bodywork* 5(4) (2012): 15–20.

22 Harper, B., 'Birth, bath, and beyond: The science and safety of water immersion during labor and birth.' *Journal of Perinatal Education* 23(3) (2014): 124–34.

23 Ullman R., Smith, L. A., Burns, E., Mori, R. and Dowswell, T., 'The use of opioid intramuscular and intravenous pain relieving drugs in labour.' *Cochrane Database of Systematic Reviews* 9 (2010).

24 Brocklehurst, P. *et al.*, (Birthplace in England Collaborative Group), 'Perinatal and maternal outcomes by planned place of birth for healthy women with low risk pregnancies: The Birthplace in England national prospective cohort study.' *British Medical Journal* 343 (2011). Available at www.npeu.ox.ac.uk/birthplace. Accessed on 29 January 2016.

25 National Institute for Health and Care Excellence (NICE), *Intrapartum Care for Healthy Women and Babies* (NICE Guidelines [CG190], December 2014). Available at www.nice.org.uk/guidance/cg190. Accessed on 3 January 2016.

26 Brocklehurst, P. *et al.*, (Birthplace in England Collaborative Group), 'Perinatal and maternal outcomes by planned place of birth for healthy women with low risk pregnancies: The Birthplace in England national prospective cohort study.' *British Medical Journal* 343 (2011). Available at www.npeu.ox.ac.uk/birthplace. Accessed on 29 January 2016.

27 Brocklehurst, P. *et al.*, (Birthplace in England Collaborative Group), 'Perinatal and maternal outcomes by planned place of birth for healthy women with low risk pregnancies: The Birthplace in England national prospective cohort study.' *British Medical Journal* 343 (2011). Available at www.npeu.ox.ac.uk/birthplace. Accessed on 29 January 2016.

28 National Institute for Health and Care Excellence (NICE), *Intrapartum Care for Healthy Women and Babies* (NICE Guidelines [CG190], December 2014). Available at www.nice.org.uk/guidance/cg190. Accessed on 3 January 2016.

29 Alfirevic, Z., Devane, D. and Gyte, G. M. L., 'Continuous cardiotocography (CTG) as a form of electronic fetal monitoring (EFM) for fetal assessment during labour.' *Cochrane Database of Systematic Reviews* 4 (2007).

30 Boyle, Maureen (ed.), *Emergencies around Childbirth: A Handbook for Midwives* (2nd edn) (Radcliffe Publishing, 2011).

31 Boyle, Maureen (ed.), *Emergencies around Childbirth: A Handbook for Midwives* (2nd edn) (Radcliffe Publishing, 2011), p. 126.

32 Cohain, J. S., 'Management of true shoulder dystocia at attended home birth.' *Midwifery Today* 103 (2012): 28–9, 69.

33 Weeks, A. D. *et al.*, 'Innovation in immediate neonatal care: Development of the Bedside Assessment, Stabilisation and Initial Cardiorespiratory Support (BASICS) Trolley.' *BMJ Innovations* 1(2) (2015): 53–58.

34 Palme-Kilander, C., 'Methods of resuscitation in low Apgar score in newborn infants – a national survey.' *Acta Paediatrica* 81 (1992): 739–44.

35 Hutchon, David, 'Ventilation before umbilical cord clamping improves physiological transition at birth or "Umbilical cord clamping before ventilation is established destabilizes physiological transition at birth".' *Frontiers in Pediatrics* 3(29) (2015).

36 Boyle, Maureen (ed.), *Emergencies around Childbirth: A Handbook for Midwives* (2nd edn) (Radcliffe Publishing, 2011), p. 55.

37 Brocklehurst, P. *et al.*, (Birthplace in England Collaborative Group), 'Perinatal and maternal outcomes by planned place of birth for healthy women with low risk pregnancies: The Birthplace in England national prospective cohort study.' *British Medical Journal* 343 (2011). Available at www.npeu.ox.ac.uk/birthplace. Accessed on 29 January 2016.

38 Frye, Anne, *Holistic Midwifery (Volume 1): Care During Pregnancy* (Lady's Press, 1995).

39 Jukic, A. M., Baird, D. D., Weinberg, C.,R., McConnaughey, D. R. and Wilcox, A. J., 'Length of human pregnancies can vary naturally by as much as five weeks.' (Oxford University Press/ ScienceDaily, 6 August 2013).

40 Dunsworth, Holly, 'Metabolic hypothesis for human altriciality.' *Proceedings of the National Academy of Sciences* 109 (38) (2012).

41 Boulvain, M., Stan, C. M. and Irion, O., 'Membrane sweeping for induction of labour.' *Cochrane Database of Systematic Reviews* (1) (2005).

42 National Institute for Health and Care Excellence (NICE), *Inducing Labour* (NICE Guidelines [CG70], July 2008).

43 Gülmezoglu, M., Crowther, C. A., Middleton, P. and Heatley, E., 'Induction of labour for improving birth outcomes for women at

or beyond term.' *Cochrane Database of Systematic Reviews* (6) (2012).

44 Horne, A., 'Postdates information.' Available at www.homebirth. org.uk. Accessed on 2 January 2016.

45 Menticoglou, Savas M. and Hall, Philip F., 'Routine induction of labour at 41 weeks gestation: Nonsensus consensus.' *BJOG: an International Journal of Obstetrics and Gynaecology* 109 (2002): 485–91.

46 Kloosterman, G. J., 'The universal aspects of childbirth: Human birth as a socio-psychosomatic paradigm.' *Journal of Psychosomatic Obstetrics and Gynecology* 1(1) (1982): 35–41. Available at www. tandfonline.com. Accessed on 29 January 2016. Quote on page 189 reprinted by permission of the publisher (Taylor and Francis Ltd.).

47 Trevathan, W. R., 'An Evolutionary Perspective on Authoritative Knowledge about Birth.' In Robbie E. Davis-Floyd and Caroline Sargent (eds) *Childbirth and Authoritative Knowledge: Cross Cultural Perspectives* (University of California Press, 1997).

48 Morgan, E., *The Descent of Woman* (Stein and Day, 1972).

49 Trevathan, W. R., 'An Evolutionary Perspective on Authoritative Knowledge about Birth.' In Robbie E. Davis-Floyd and Caroline Sargent (eds) *Childbirth and Authoritative Knowledge: Cross Cultural Perspectives* (University of California Press, 1997).

50 Trevathan, W. R., 'An Evolutionary Perspective on Authoritative Knowledge about Birth.' In Robbie E. Davis-Floyd and Caroline Sargent (eds) *Childbirth and Authoritative Knowledge: Cross Cultural Perspectives* (University of California Press, 1997).

51 'Long-held theory on human gestation refuted: Mother's metabolism, not birth canal size, limits gestation.' (University of Rhode Island/ScienceDaily, 27 August 2012).

52 Dunsworth, H., 'Metabolic hypothesis for human altriciality.' *Proceedings of the National Academy of Sciences* 109(38) (2012).

53 ScienceDaily, 'Long-held theory on human gestation refuted: Mother's metabolism, not birth canal size, limits gestation.' (University of Rhode Island/ScienceDaily, 27 August 2012). Available at http://www.sciencedaily.com/releases/2012/08/120827152037.htm. Accessed on 30 January 2016.

54 Limburg, A., Smulders, B. and Rees, S., *Women Giving Birth* (Celestial Arts Publishing, 1992).

55 Gupta, J., Hofmeyr, G. and Smith, R., 'Position for women during second stage of labour for women without epidural anaesthesia.' *Cochrane Database of Systematic Reviews* 1 (2004).

56 Limburg, Astrid and Smulders, Beatrijs, *Women Giving Birth* (Celestial Arts Publishing, 1992).

57 Tew, Marjorie, *Safer Childbirth? A Critical History of Maternity Care* (Free Association Books, 1990, 1998).

58 Davis, A., *Choice, Policy and Practice in Maternity Care Since 1948* (History & Policy papers, 2013).

59 Ministry of Health, *Report of the Committee of Enquiry into the Cost of the National Health Service* (Chairman C. Guillebaud) (HMSO, 1959).

60 Tew, Marjorie, *Safer Childbirth? A Critical History of Maternity Care* (Free Association Books, 1990, 1998).

61 Ministry of Health, *Domiciliary Midwifery and Maternity Bed Needs: The Report of the Standing Maternity and Midwifery Advisory Committee* (Sub-committee Chairman J. Peel) (HMSO, 1970).

62 Beech, B. A. and Robinson, J., *Ultrasound? Unsound* (AIMS, 1994).

63 Maternity Services Advisory Committee, *Maternity Care in Action. Part 2 Care During Childbirth (Intrapartum Care): A Guide to Good Practice and a Plan for Action* (HMSO, 1984).

64 Tew, Marjorie, *Safer Childbirth? A Critical History of Maternity Care* (Free Association Books, 1998).

65 Department of Health, *Changing Childbirth: Report of the Expert Maternity Group* (Chairman Lady Julia Cumberledge) (HMSO, 1993).

66 Tew, Marjorie, *Safer Childbirth? A Critical History of Maternity Care* (Free Association Books, 1998).

67 Department of Health (DoH), *Maternity Matters: Choice, Access and Continuity of Care in a Safe Service.* (DoH, 2007).

68 National Childbirth Trust (NCT), *NCT Policy Briefing: Choice of Place of Birth* (NCT, 2011). Available at www.nct.org.uk/sites/default/files/related_documents/MS13%20Choice%20of%20place%20of%20birth_0.pdf. Accessed on 2 January 2016.

69 Flint, C. and Poulangeris, P., *The 'Know your Midwife' Report* (South West Thames Regional Health Authority and the Wellington Foundation, 1987).

70 Tew, Marjorie, *Safer Childbirth? A Critical History of Maternity Care* (Free Association Books, 1998).

71 Tew, Marjorie, *Safer Childbirth? A Critical History of Maternity Care* (Free Association Books, 1998).

72 Brocklehurst, P. *et al.*, (Birthplace in England Collaborative Group), 'Perinatal and maternal outcomes by planned place of birth for healthy women with low risk pregnancies: The Birthplace in England national prospective cohort study.' *British Medical Journal* 343 (2011). Available at www.npeu.ox.ac.uk/birthplace. Accessed on 29 January 2016.

73 National Institute for Health and Care Excellence (NICE), *Intrapartum Care for Healthy Women and Babies* (NICE Guidelines [CG190], December 2014). Available at www.nice.org.uk/guidance/cg190. Accessed on 3 January 2016.

74 Association of Radical Midwives, *New Vision for Maternity Care* (2013). Available at www.midwifery.org.uk. Accessed on 2 January 2016.

75 Byrom, S. and Downe, S. (eds), *The Roar Behind the Silence* (Pinter and Martin, 2015).

76 Downe, S (ed.), *Normal Childbirth Evidence and Debate* (2nd edn) (Elsevier, 2008).

77 Arms, S., *Immaculate Deception II: Myth, Magic and Birth* (Celestial Arts, 1996).

78 Kirkup, B., *The Report of the Morecombe Bay Investigation* (The Stationery Office, 2015).

79 Francis, R., QC, *Report of the Mid Staffordshire NHS Foundation Trust Public Enquiry* (The Stationery Office, February 2013).

80 National Institute for Health and Care Excellence (NICE), *Intrapartum Care for Healthy Women and Babies* (NICE Guidelines [CG190], December 2014). Available at www.nice.org.uk/guidance/cg190. Accessed on 3 January 2016.

81 National Institute for Health and Care Excellence (NICE), *Intrapartum Care for Healthy Women and Babies* (NICE Guidelines [CG190], December 2014). Available at www.nice.org.uk/guidance/cg190. Accessed on 3 January 2016.

82 Brocklehurst, P. *et al.*, (Birthplace in England Collaborative Group), 'Perinatal and maternal outcomes by planned place of birth for healthy women with low risk pregnancies: The Birthplace

in England national prospective cohort study.' *British Medical Journal* 343 (2011). Available at www.npeu.ox.ac.uk/birthplace. Accessed on 29 January 2016.

83 National Perinatal Birthplace Epidemiology (NPEU) Unit, Birthplace in England Research Programme. Available at www. npeu.ox.ac.uk/birthplace. Accessed on 29 January 2016.

84 Schroeder, L., Petrou, S., Patel, N., Hollowell, J., Puddicombe, D., Redshaw, M., *et al.* 'Birthplace cost-effectiveness analysis of planned place of birth: individual level analysis. Birthplace in England Research Programme. Final Report Part 5 (NIHR Service Delivery and Organisation programme, 2011). Available at www. nets.nihr.ac.uk/__data/assets/pdf_file/0007/84949/FR5-08-1604-140.pdf. Accessed on 29 January 2016.

85 National Perinatal Birthplace Epidemiology (NPEU) Unit, Birthplace in England Research Programme. Available at www. npeu.ox.ac.uk/downloads/files/birthplace/Birthplace-Q-A.pdf Accessed on 29 January 2016.

86 Hollowell J., Rowe R., Townend J., Knight M., Li Y., Linsell L., et al. 'The Birthplace in England National Prospective Cohort Study: further analyses to enhance policy and service delivery decision-making for planned place of birth' Health Serv Deliv Res 2015; 3(36). Available at: https://www.npeu.ox.ac.uk/birthplace/birth-place-follow-on-study. Accessed 28 February 2016.

87 National Institute for Health and Care Excellence (NICE), *Intrapartum Care for Healthy Women and Babies* (NICE Guidelines [CG190], December 2014). Available at www.nice.org.uk/guid-ance/cg190. Accessed 28 February 2016.

Index

Index

273

Index